YOU WERE CREATED FOR GREATNESS

A PHILOSOPHY ON WHOLENESS

2ND EDITION

Jackson Hale

YOU WERE CREATED FOR GREATNESS 2nd edition

ISBN: 979-8-218-11412-1

Cover Designed by Maja Kapunovic

A Message to the Reader

This is a book of revival. Reviving what was lost, what was broken, what was stolen, and the God-given potential deep within you. I burn with a Christ-centered focus to help you run this race as a Believer with health, consistency, passion, and joy for the Kingdom.

So, I call the Church for change. I call the Church to impact the world like never before through the power and the love of the Holy Spirit gifted inside of you. Yet, we must examine ourselves. We must look at where we are at physically, mentally, and spiritually, and ask ourselves, are we ready?

Are we ready to be all in for the things of God beyond our wildest imagination, through complete health, freedom, and sonship to the Father?

Yes, it will take time. It will take effort. But you are chosen. You are set apart to make the difference in this world that it so desperately needs—a generation looking beyond itself, and humble enough to *exude* Jesus in every area of their life.

This is *complete* abandonment of the worldly desires and culture of this world for something bigger than yourself.

Greatness.

You are called. This book is for you. And it starts now.

Welcome to My Philosophy on Wholeness.

Gratitude

To all who helped, encouraged, and enlightened me along the way, I could not have written this without you. Thank you to my mother and father, my sister, and my brothers and sisters in Christ: Clarence, Tyler, Jamal, Natalie, Tom, Max, Dillon, Carlos, Nick, Becca, Paul, Bryan, Dave, Chad, Julie, Joe, Cassidy, Jeff, Hal, Dan, Shawn, Craig, Mike, Cynthia, Pastor Joel, Brianna, Alyssa, Amanda, Andrea, Dominick, and Professor Crowell.

With the second edition I have taken the time to add new material, expanding my thoughts and update my current focus around the heart of the 360wellness ministry: Revival. I thank God for the opportunity to present you these next pages, and I give Him all the glory.

I have poured all I know and believe into this book. I pray it produces the good fruit I intend to plant in doing so. Throughout the total seven chapters, there will be practical tips along with a twenty-question holistic assessment at the end. This is for an opportunity to explore your current health and wellness, so I encourage you to bring a notebook along for the journey and journal what you feel led to. Thank you for reading, it is truly a blessing; I am honored.

TABLE OF CONTENTS

Introduction

"But this is not how it is among you; instead, whoever wishes to become great among you must be your servant, and whoever wishes to be first and most important among you must be slave of all. For even the Son of Man did not come to be served, but to serve, and to give His life as a ransom for many."

Mark 10:43-45 AMP

Greatness isn't about money. It isn't about skill. It isn't about the number of people you reach. *It's about the depth of impact one makes in the lives of others*. Through Christ-centered wellness, you can consistently maximize your impact in this world. It will take time, effort, persistence, and focus, but you have what it takes. After all, you were made in His image.

Now that you host the Holy Spirit as a Believer, you have everything you need. God can use you for His glory. Yet, you have free choice to either cultivate a healthy environment in your life where you can be used to your full potential or squander the opportunity by giving into the temptations and distractions of this world.

So, you must ask yourself. Which will it be?

Through greatness you will achieve much. Your actions, however, must be tactical and intentional in this world as a Believer. It's needed even more now than ever to be sober minded and full of love in the freedom Christ has given us.

God's hope and intention for you is to live your best life for His glory, impacting those in your sphere of influence through His love and power. *Our potential is in Him.*

You have a path. You have a destiny. But will you say, *"yes"* to a life of wholeness and run your best?

My goal with this book is to pour out everything I have learned, my heart, and what I believe in as a faith-based wellness professional. This is something I now know I need for my own life. God has put it on my heart to write out my belief on personal wholeness, and I have written these pages to piece together what I have found to be essential for consistent health in my life. Please know I am walking this out daily, and I am with you.

I am no expert, doctor, or pastor, but what I do carry is a burning passion to see the Body of Christ consistently walk with confidence, power, and love in the Spirit. I am talking about working toward consistent transformation into who He has created you to be.

Physical health is not the end-all-be-all. Through personal experience, and helping clients along their own journey, I strongly believe this to be true. There is a deeper health a person needs, and as a Christian myself, I've noticed the Church—His body—needs as well. A holistic health.

I have learned in my own life that, as a Believer, you must be diligent and intentional in how you take care of your body, mind, and spirit as you seek to abide, grow, and remain consistent in your walk with God.

You are a complex human being with a great destiny through Christ. However, you have free will. There is opposition, along with many distractions and false truths in this world constantly pulling you away from your potential. This book will teach you how to build healthy stability in your life, cut through the distractions this world so tangibly holds, and empower your best self to unlock the God-given potential within.

Again, through greatness, you will achieve much. Each of your dreams may look different, but no matter where you are in life, you have value, and you can have a positive impact in the lives of others.

It's not what you do but how you

do it that makes a difference.

God can use you wherever He plants you. But in order to consistently steward your best you must cultivate and set the foundation for greatness. This is what I call true wellness, or "wholeness" in your life. Amen.

You must realize the Gospel is a holistic message. It brings everlasting life for all who will drink the water of Christ.

John 4:13-14 AMP, *"Jesus answered her, 'Everyone who drinks this water will be thirsty again. But whoever drinks the water that I give him will never be thirsty again. But the water that I give him will become in him a spring of water [satisfying his thirst for God] welling up [continually flowing, bubbling within him] to eternal life.'"*

By letting it seep into every part of your life, you will transform into a new creation.

The old is gone. The new is living. And all that held you back in the past is now nothing but a memory.

> Hebrews 8:11-12 AMP, *"And it will not be [necessary] for each one to teach his fellow citizen, Or each one his brother, saying, 'Know [by experience, have knowledge of] the Lord,'*
>
> *For all will know [Me by experience and have knowledge of] Me, From the least to the greatest of them. For I will be merciful and gracious toward their wickedness, And I will remember their sins no more."*

When you step into this truth and trust the scriptures, your identity will begin to come into view. *Your true identity.* First and foremost, that you are a child of God.

Through this truth, you can begin to love in opposition of the world's selfish and destructive culture. From the way you engage in relationship to others, to the way you eat, to the way you approach health and even fitness.

My mission is to bring you into a place of realization of who you are, what you are worth, and the potential of impact you carry for God's kingdom.

This deep, Christ-centered, holistic take on wellness is my passion for all whom I meet through the Church, on the street, or connect with throughout the pages of this book. You need to know and remember we all have purpose in Christ; we all have reason for being here on earth. Life is a journey to walk out this truth, and I will help optimize it.

So, it starts here— building a foundation of greatness through true health and wellness: a foundation that is Christ-centered and empowers you to be your best, whole self, so you can give your best to those around you who need it most.

This is what it's all about and what Christ focused on daily. Although I struggle too, personally, I feel most alive when I am giving, helping, or tending to someone in need.

> Acts 20:35 AMP, *"In everything I showed you [by example] that by working hard in this way you must help the weak and remember the words of the Lord Jesus, that He Himself said, 'It is more blessed [and brings greater joy] to give than to receive.'"*

I may not always feel like it, but I know it is better to give than receive. Think about the last time you reached out to help someone in need. How did it feel?

Selfless giving is a gift in and of itself. Part of these pages will help you get to a place where you can come from this spiritual abundance of giving not just needing, the way scripture has called you to live and love.

My focus in all this centers around two principles: *prevention* and *consistency*.

Preventing the things the world cultivates, such as pain, sickness, disease, obesity, depression, anxiety, and so on. Many of the things experienced today are unnecessary and can be prevented by bringing awareness and tending to the right areas in need. Not all, but most.

With less of this in your life you can begin to come from a place of consistent outreach to those in need.

You can begin to look

forward and not down.

Yet, I know and understand this is not the way the world works, and sometimes, it can even seem like everything is against this kind of living (which I believe it is).

Secondly, I want you to know that you were built for consistency. Consistently loving, living, praying, and walking in the Spirit. This is the goal, and I have a strong conviction to help you rise to the occasion.

I did not, however, start my wellness journey with this conviction. In 2014, I had an idea for a company I call 360wellness. I began this health and wellness startup with a simple Instagram profile focused on corrective exercise, nutrition, and preventative health while simultaneously discovering my passions junior year of college.

As I continued into my senior year, I gained experience in the healthcare industry working under an amazing team of physical therapists as a Physical Therapy Aide.

Through my work, I connected with the two lead therapists, Nadar and Mary, who were both Christian and had come from Egypt looking to start a life in America. Where over many years, they developed this successful business named Agape Physical Therapy ("*Agape*" happens to mean *unconditional love*).

God's love.

I will never forget the day I applied for an internship at Agape. As I was driving by and hesitant to apply for an internship position, something pulled on my heart (which I later learned was a nudge from the Holy Spirit).

I ended up pulling a U-turn and going inside. This ultimately led me to work with them for an entire year while I finished my time at Azusa Pacific University in Southern California. I learned amazing concepts and applications in the rehab field that I still use with patients today.

However, I felt there was something missing in this kind of care, and I was hungry to bridge the gap. While I was involved in my internship, I learned two things:

The first is I was empathetic toward my clients, and it broke my heart. Every time I would work with someone in pain from post-surgery or an injury, I wished there had been a way to prevent it.

It seemed like 80 percent of the cases coming through could have been prevented if caught early.

The second is the healthcare system unfortunately made it difficult for the patient and the provider to do what they needed to do for full recovery (along with prevention of further pain/injury). There just wasn't enough time or money to solve the issues at hand.

As I graduated, I continued my journey to San Diego and found my true relationship with God through multiple experiences that I cannot deny. From walking into a revival service and feeling the presence of God, to flying with a missionary team to Africa and seeing God heal hundreds of children through our hands.

I recognized the power of faith in

Jesus Christ and the healing, health,

and peace that comes with it.

Most importantly I experienced what a true, intimate relationship with Him produces. Life.

There are many things available to us that provide a temporary peace, but through faith and relationship with God, there's an opportunity for something deeper, something that is true and lasting.

Jesus is the missing piece in wellness that very few professionals can and are emphasizing in their model of client care. I want things to change. This application to your life satisfies and allows you to graduate to a place of Godly leadership and love, founding characteristics of greatness.

This view has led me to continually evolve 360wellness, as the concepts have with it. I always had a foundation of preventative health and well-being in the beginning with massage, exercise, nutrition, and mindfulness being the founding business concepts in 2016. I had quickly learned what my fitness and therapy clients needed most for a balanced life.

But as you can see, time went on, and God began to lead me toward this Christ-centered focus on healthcare. Christ is our cornerstone, and without Him, we have nothing.

> John 15:5 *"I am the Vine; you are the branches. The one who remains in Me and I in him bears much fruit, for [otherwise] apart from Me [that is, cut off from vital union with Me] you can do nothing."*

And so, my vision began to change. My passions began to change. God began to transform 360wellness and over time, it has become the way I know He intended it to be. It impacts others past the physical level, empowering all to be who they were created to be. Passionate sons and daughters of the King.

Revival.

This vision came into full view at the end of 2019, when I received a word from God going into the new year saying, *"We Will See Clearly."*

As I wrote this in the middle of the year 2020, I began to see that eyes were opening to what should be truly valued in life and the gift of life that oftentimes we forget to be grateful for.

It was and is time for change. One may say a pivot. I therefore believe in proclaiming a health that doesn't just focus on the physical and mental aspects of a person but also empower the spirit with a Christ-centered approach. This is the journey of wholeness. This is where everything flows.

> *You do not have complete health without your*
>
> *spirit being nurtured and tended to.*

My passion and calling is to bridge the gap between healthcare and faith, providing support, direction, and training for the Body of Christ, helping to maximize its impact. Imagine a holistic health care system open to God's love and Spirit, freely and openly confessing that Christ is Lord while providing elite professional care to all who will come.

This would be a place where prayer is a part of culture and the healing process, a place where you have faith-based care from working professionals who want to see you live your best life for God's glory.

This has been building inside of me, and I have a dream to one day make a global impact with 360wellness through a system capable of helping others find health and wholeness across the globe. This would cultivate a culture of helping to empower churches, third-world communities, the less-fortunate in America, the homeless, and the broken.

Does this sound like a lot? Let me reiterate the foundation.

I realize the importance and power in integrating holistic health of the body, mind, and spirit. I also know your potential. This way of living will maximize and give clarity to your walk of faith in our complex efforts to become whole.

I look at *wholeness* as, "a state of working toward health in not just the physical, but also the mental and spiritual."

This is a continual process and is a precursor to what I call "true wellness," or deep health. As you work toward this kind of foundation, you can set up God (and the Holy Spirit) to be most active in your life— seeing clearly, walking in purity (of all kinds), and limiting the distractions of this world.

The concept is in addition to God's grace, you will have to take diligent, intentional, organized action to be at your best. For faith without works is dead.

> James 2:26 AMP, *"For just as the [human] body without the spirit is dead, so faith without works [of obedience] is also dead."*

Within the Body of Christ, there is a need to become more proactive with our holistic health, to live with prevention in mind.

To be proactive is defined as, *"(of a person or action) creating or controlling a situation by causing something to happen rather than responding to it after it has happened"* (Oxford Dictionaries, 2020).

On paper, maintaining this kind of holistic health is easy:

Stay active, eat your veggies, build connection with others, pray, read scripture, serve, and so on. If you are being realistic however, things— kids, injury, pain, lack of motivation, distractions, and other priorities (or idols) — get in the way.

Now, before we move forward and walk through *the concept* of my philosophy on wholeness, I would like to call out and identify some of the reasons and/or *lies* that keep us from building a foundation of true wellness in our lives.

1. Knowledge

> You might not be truly aware of the benefits of self-care, exercise, sound nutrition, sleep, stress management, prayer, and the practices alike. Knowledge (AND action) is power.

2. Support

It's hard to do it alone and that's ok. That's normal. All of us need support, direction, and encouragement throughout life. The same applies to your health. I believe everyone should have a coach, mentor, or partner to help maximize their potential.

Seek those around you whom you can trust. Tell them your story and your goals. This can keep you accountable and push you when you're feeling down. You never know, they may even be motivated by you and want to start a connect group.

3. *"It's vanity"*

During this day and age, the fitness industry sexualizes health. Many people want to look better to impress others (or themselves), gaining a kind of confidence and self-worth from body image.

But that isn't what this book is about. I'd like to say there are always two ways of doing things. They both may look the same, but it's all about intention. Where the heart is, is what matters most.

> Matthew 15:18 AMP, *"But whatever [word] comes out of the mouth comes from the heart, and this is what defiles and dishonors the man."*

Health is much deeper than the physical. And the good thing about tending to yours? The outside will always reflect the care you do on the inside.

The more you care for your body with

pure intentions, the more you'll notice

the true "you" starting to show.

This has always reminded me of Jesus preaching, *"seek first the kingdom of God"* (Matthew 6:33).

First tend to yourself from the inside-out with righteousness and purity and all you are looking for will come into place. There's no need to strive.

Listen, we all have a certain body type— the way God made us. The more you change your mindset from how the world views health and fitness and your negative thoughts, the more you can be realistic and content with your body, tending to yourself as a temple of God, not something to disgrace.

4. *"I'm not good enough/worth it"*

This is a lie. The devil is a liar, and the fact that you are alive and breathing today shows you have purpose; you may just need to find it.

If you think no one else believes in you, I do. I trust you are on to great things for the sake of the Kingdom and others if you allow yourself to believe.

Yet, you must know that consistency in life starts with self-care. If you pour into others without pouring into yourself, how can you be your best? How can you give your best? Perspective is everything. And You. Are. Worth. It.

Believe me, it's not always about how you feel. *Sometimes you just have to walk by faith and watch it grow.*

We must begin to see everyone's potential reflected in the image of God. This is where unconditional love begins— a love for God, and others because first and foremost we were made in His image. You are a Son or Daughter. Your potential is everything, and Jesus was sent to restore that. He loved you first (1 John 4:9).

Do you not know who you are?

5. *"I don't have time"*

This may feel true. We all experience overwhelming pressure from work, responsibility, daily tasks, family, and personal goals, but it's always a matter of priority. Time will always be limited, and it cannot be renewed.

You must decide to make the time,

no matter how small it may be.

Even just a few minutes daily, or 10 percent effort, can yield huge results in the long run when working toward your goals. To maximize your potential, it's all about prioritizing and staying consistent.

Find your marathon pace!

6. *"It's just not my thing"*

That's fair. Taking weekly spa days, working out in the gym seven days a week, becoming an ordained minister, and prepping organic cooked meals with your personal chef may not be realistic. You may not even have an interest. And that's ok.

There is no perfect route or process here. You just need to find what you enjoy and be real. You can do your best with what God has given you. The beautiful thing is God meets you where you are at, giving you more to manage when you can handle it.

Matthew 25:29 AMP, *"For to everyone who has [and values his blessings and gifts from God, and has used them wisely], more will be given, and [he will be richly supplied so that] he will have an abundance; but from the one who does not have [because he has ignored or disregarded his blessings and gifts from God], even what he does have will be taken away."*

7. Filling a void

Lastly, you may use certain lifestyle habits like fast food, social media, alcohol, or caffeine as a filler (I know I have). But let me encourage and remind you this:

Only God will satisfy and sustain your insatiable

need for love, wholeness, and peace.

He is with you, and you are not alone in this. If you can have faith to break through the fog, even for a moment, reaching out to God for strength, building healthy habits and finding support (in the body, mind, and spirit) can provide the fulfillment you truly seek.

Acts 2:21 AMP, *" 'And it shall be that everyone who calls upon the name of the Lord [invoking, adoring, and worshiping the Lord Jesus] shall be saved (rescued spiritually).' "*

No matter what, the foundation of health stays the same. Focus on your health and understand it because you matter, you will be your best, and you will feel your best throughout this journey we call life. No matter what trials the world brings, or what opportunities you have to pour into others, you will be making an impact in people's lives and in God's kingdom wherever He plants you.

So, don't believe the lies.

This book is a philosophy on wholeness; a philosophy on how you can heal from and prevent the world's negative impact on the body, mind, and spirit. It's also a solution to help you revive your spirit and maximize the God-given potential within so you can walk as an influencer in this world—As a leader, not a follower, for the glory of God.

In the next seven chapters, I have laid out a healthy, integrated foundation of wholeness for your body, mind, and spirit. God wants you to shine, and I call out the gold in you!

Remember, everyone's greatness may look different, but it's up to you and your perspective to make the most of what you have in this world, aiming to be your best.

This is a race. Your life matters. And you were created for greatness.

> 1 Corinthians 9:24-27 AMP, *"Do you not know that in a race all the runners run [their very best to win], but only one receives the prize?*
>
> *Run [your race] in such a way that you may seize the prize and make it yours! Now every athlete who [goes into training and] competes in the games is disciplined and exercises self-control in all things. They do it to win a crown that withers, but we [do it to receive] an imperishable [crown that cannot wither].*
>
> *Therefore I do not run without a definite goal; I do not flail around like one beating the air [just shadow boxing]. But [like a boxer] I strictly discipline my body and make it my slave, so that, after I have preached [the gospel] to others, I myself will not somehow be disqualified [as unfit for service]."*

Reflect

Consider the 7 reasons/lies that might be keeping you from building a true foundation of wellness in your life.

Which one do you find yourself thinking about most often?

How would your life look differently if you were free from that belief/obstacle?

Chapter I – The Concept

"For physical training is of some value, but godliness (spiritual training) is of value in everything and in every way, since it holds promise for the present life and for the life to come."

1 Timothy 4:8 AMP

In a world of pain, sickness, and disease, something needs to change. We can no longer go on just getting by. There must be action. There must be change. As the Church we must become serious about our wellness so we can consistently live in the fullness of God's plan for our life, accomplishing all that He has for us.

Wellness is not limited to just your

physical body: it expands into your mental,

emotional, and spiritual self.

This can best be explained through the biopsychosocial model, which considers multiple aspects of your life as keys to wellness. These include biological (such as age), psychological (such as mental health), and sociological (such as environment or social support) factors. I would also add "spiritual health" to this list, but more on that later.

Time and time again, people fall to unnecessary pain, addiction, depression, lack of motivation and purpose, yet you are called to greatness. Whatever this looks like to you, as a Believer, you should come from a place of abundance and rest to help those in need along your path.

You are truly called to give.

> Acts 20:35 AMP, *"In everything I showed you [by example] that by working hard in this way you must help the weak and remember the words of the Lord Jesus, that He Himself said, 'It is more blessed [and brings greater joy] to give than to receive.'"*

But how can you truly give consistently with love without first becoming *whole* yourself? From a foundational, personal point of view, I want to empower you to walk in daily wholeness, so that you, the Church (Body of Christ), can reach out with selfless love and impact those in need around you.

The following examples are related to the *flesh*, or your selfish human nature, and can leave you in a box focused on *self*, whether you realize it or not.

I call them "distractions".

- Pain
- Sickness
- Disease
- Depression
- Anxiety
- Fear
- Obesity

Now, I'd like to touch on "obesity". I am not by any means talking about those who are naturally different than the status quo of "fit." God has made all of mankind with different shapes, sizes, and metabolisms, so don't let anyone tell you otherwise.

That is a lie from the pit of hell, and I bind and rebuke in the name of Jesus Christ any insecurity or self-doubt regarding body image to those reading this page.

God loves you so much. Do not believe anything else.

> Romans 8:38-39 AMP, *"For I am convinced [and continue to be convinced—beyond any doubt] that neither death, nor life, nor angels, nor principalities, nor things present and threatening, nor things to come, nor powers, nor height, nor depth, nor any other created thing, will be able to separate us from the [unlimited] love of God, which is in Christ Jesus our Lord."*

If you are struggling with your weight, don't agree with anything else!

What I am referring to when I say obesity, is when you overeat and begin to weigh beyond your natural weight. This lifestyle can become harmful not only to your physical body and mind (heart, hormone, and mental health) but also to your spirit, as it deals with feeding the "flesh" and can lead to other distractions mentioned above.

We must be incredibly careful of the fine line between enjoying our freedom and gluttony (over-indulgence), which is rarely discussed in the Church. I will discuss this further in Chapter 4, Nutrition.

So, these seven distractions may be common or even "normal," but as a child of God, you are not called to these things (especially when a majority can be prevented). As part of the Body of Christ, you are called to health, life, and dominion, using these things to focus on others, dying to self, and picking up your cross daily to follow Jesus. It seems almost contradicting, yet it is a truly balanced way of life.

Genesis 1:26 AMP, *"Then God said, 'Let Us (Father, Son, Holy Spirit) make man in Our image, according to Our likeness [not physical, but a spiritual personality and moral likeness]; and let them have complete authority over the fish of the sea, the birds of the air, the cattle, and over the entire earth, and over everything that creeps and crawls on the earth.'"*

Luke 9:23 AMP, *"And He was saying to them all, 'If anyone wishes to follow Me [as My disciple], he must deny himself [set aside selfish interests], and take up his cross daily [expressing a willingness to endure whatever may come] and follow Me [believing in Me, conforming to My example in living and, if need be, suffering or perhaps dying because of faith in Me].'"*

Luke 4:18 AMP, *"THE SPIRIT OF THE LORD IS UPON ME (the Messiah), because He has anointed Me to preach the good news to the poor. He has sent Me to announce release (pardon, forgiveness) TO THE CAPTIVES, and recovery of sight to the blind, to set free those who are oppressed (downtrodden, bruised, crushed by tragedy)."*

Jesus sets free those who are oppressed. You're not called to sit in your room and be "Godly." You're called to go out into the world and make an impact (Matthew 28:29). The journey will not be easy but who ever said it would be, or should be? The influence of this world is doing everything in its power to stop your true greatness from manifesting.

The flesh, the world, and the devil, with all their confusion, distractions, and temptations are in direct opposition to what you are called to walk in—the Spirit (Galatians 5). You must be alert and do everything in your best interest for the Kingdom of God (which is righteousness, peace, and joy in the Spirit).

Romans 14:17 NASB, *"For the kingdom of God is not eating and drinking, but righteousness and peace and joy in the Holy Spirit."*

Ultimately, what you must realize is this life is not about you and it never has been. Love God. Love others. I promise in this, you will find true freedom and joy, taking the focus off yourself.

Galatians 5:13 AMP, *"For you, my brothers, were called to freedom; only do not let your freedom become an opportunity for the sinful nature (worldliness, selfishness), but through love serve and seek the best for one another."*

John 8:31-32 AMP, *So Jesus was saying to the Jews who had believed Him, "If you abide in My word [continually obeying My teachings and living in accordance with them, then] you are truly My disciples. And you will know the truth [regarding salvation], and the truth will set you free [from the penalty of sin]."*

Matthew 10:39 AMP, *"Whoever finds his life [in this world] will [eventually] lose it [through death], and whoever loses his life [in this world] for My sake will find it [that is, life with Me for all eternity]."*

Yet, you still must value yourself as a temple of God, know His love for you, and obey God's Word.

1 Corinthians 3:16 AMP, *"Do you not know and understand that you [the church] are the temple of God, and that the Spirit of God dwells [permanently] in you [collectively and individually]?"*

Romans 8:38-39 AMP, *"For I am convinced [and continue to be convinced—beyond any doubt] that neither death, nor life, nor angels, nor principalities, nor things present and threatening, nor things to come, nor powers, nor height, nor depth, nor any other created thing, will be able to separate us from the [unlimited] love of God, which is in Christ Jesus our Lord."*

2 Corinthians 6:16 AMP, *"What agreement is there between the temple of God and idols? For we are the temple of the living God; just as God said: 'I WILL DWELL IN THEM AND WALK AMONG THEM; AND I WILL BE THEIR GOD, AND THEY SHALL BE MY PEOPLE.'"*

You may now be asking yourself, "Ok, how do I begin to do this?" The following pages will explain and walk you through each concept of 360wellness to promote this way of wholeness. This is what I believe makes up a solid foundation for your life of greatness as a Believer.

Know that I am with you throughout this journey and only have your best interests in mind. What God has spoken directly to my heart is, "Heal My People." I know He is talking about you. The Church. God's people. His chosen.

There is brokenness and hurt in the Body of

Christ, but I call for restoration.

Not for personal gain, as I am not doing this for money or attention but solely from the heart through what God has taught me on my own journey (and is continuing to teach me). It has been eight years since the first vision of 360wellness, and it continues to evolve as God leads this fluid organization.

Again, the Gospel is a holistic message, and I must integrate this into what I do. I believe with all my heart that the body affects the mind/spirit and vice versa, yet rarely do we apply intention and change to this.

This mentality has brought me to start a ministry that focuses on the restoration and revival of God's people and all who will come. At the end of the day, my foundation in all of this is prevention and consistency. In this day and age, being prevention-focused and consistent with our actions is *essential* to being steady as a Believer.

We must begin to act against our sedentary jobs, quick result mindsets ("microwave mentality"), lust of food and drink, high stress environments, self-centeredness, and the distractions of pain, sickness, and disease that the world so easily creates.

I continue to call these things "distractions" because they can pull us away from our number one purpose: to consistently love God and others.

> Matthew 22:36-39 AMP, *"Teacher, which is the greatest commandment in the Law? And Jesus replied to him, 'YOU SHALL LOVE THE LORD YOUR GOD WITH ALL YOUR HEART, AND WITH ALL YOUR SOUL, AND WITH ALL YOUR MIND.'*

> *This is the first and greatest commandment. The second is like it, 'YOU SHALL LOVE YOUR NEIGHBOR AS YOURSELF [that is, unselfishly seek the best or higher good for others].'"*

It's hard to help or pray for someone else when you are distracted and dealing with your own "issues." Do you have to be perfect and have everything figured out? Of course not. But ultimately, you aren't called to live this kind of life.

Yes, as human beings we have in a way brought this upon ourselves: the environment we grew up in, our busy lives, incredible demands at work, and the food and drink industries are just giving us what we want. But there's the problem— *it's what we want.*

Yet, it's not entirely our fault. In some ways, we've been born into it. From the type of family we grew up with, to the fast-paced culture we live in today, we learned to adopt certain habits and mindsets.

Personally, I was raised in Texas. My family was small and simple, and taught to finish the food left on the plate. To enjoy Bluebell ice cream every chance you had, and if you were old enough (or not) to have a beer and "loosen up." Self-control and health were a second thought. This was culture.

This is culture.

Your lifestyle may look different to you now than it did in the past, but the foundations of this worldly culture are the same. And unfortunately, they do not produce good, lasting fruit. They are not centered in Christ.

Through my own experience and working with clients of every background, there is a "better way."

You can no longer carry these habits or related

ones with you into a maturing Christian life.

Notice I say maturing. As a Christian, you are called to more by regarding your body as God's temple now that you host the Holy Spirit (1 Corinthians 3:16-17). Another scripture that has been a foundation for my life and 360wellness (yet isn't discussed often in healthcare or the Church) is:

> 1 Timothy 4:8 AMP, *"For physical training is of some value, but godliness (spiritual training) is of value in everything and in every way, since it holds promise for the present life and for the life to come."*

This book is not just about taking mature action, caring for your physical and mental state. It's also about taking care of your spirit and integrating the action of faith daily into your walk as a Believer.

Most of the concepts throughout the following pages, you will know. They may be taken to a new depth, but they are used by most of us. There's one, however, that's less common.

It is the integration of health and wellness into the Christian Body—*a place where science freely meets faith.*

In the technology and progress of today, we must be proactive in healthcare, wellness, and new applications within the Church, and that's ok. As the distractions of the world and accessibility to those distractions rise, our actions must go "from glory to glory" in all areas of life.

2 Corinthians 3:17-18 AMP, *"Now the Lord is the Spirit, and where the Spirit of the Lord is, there is liberty [emancipation from bondage, true freedom]. And we all, with unveiled face, continually seeing as in a mirror the glory of the Lord, are progressively being transformed into His image from [one degree of] glory to [even more] glory, which comes from the Lord, [who is] the Spirit."*

You must begin to think and act differently to be set apart from the ways of the world. As you are continually transformed into the image of Christ, your day-to-day actions need to transform with you, all the way down to healthy, foundational wellness. We're talking "the mind of Christ."

This is stewarding well all that God has given you. Imagine if the Christian Church lived with this conviction: *That I am enough and that I can have the impact God desires in my life through tending to my wellness.* True wellness, consistently, not just in the body but also in mind and spirit.

We must move past the "old-school" way of doing things, acting by sheer will, even shaming others (or ourselves) for not keeping up or staying consistent. We need direction and new application to walk consistently in purity of the body, mind, and spirit as Believers. The worldly influence around us does not make it easy, so this holistic kind of thinking is what, I believe, true wellness boils down to.

Matthew 26:40-41 AMP, *"And He came to the disciples and found them sleeping, and said to Peter,*

'So, you men could not stay awake and keep watch with Me for one hour? Keep actively watching and praying that you may not come into temptation; the spirit is willing, but the body is weak.'"

You can no longer continue off willpower and good intentions if you want to maximize your impact, lead as a good example, and empower the lives of others as Christ commanded in this world. As a Believer, you have the Holy Spirit within you, but you must empower the Spirit to be used in your life.

You must not limit the power of God. You must not limit the Holy One of Israel. There is a choice. There's always a choice. God looks for someone to rise to the occasion but finds few.

> Matthew 22:14 AMP, *"For many are called (invited, summoned), but few are chosen."*

We become available for more opportunity by creating a temple dedicated to hosting the Lord's Spirit and living a life of purity in all areas of our life (limiting the flesh and not squandering our freedom/power, Galatians 5:13). This is foundational and essential to the Christian Body for full potential.

It's called consecration.

> 2 Timothy 2:20-21 AMP, *"Now in a large house there are not only vessels and objects of gold and silver, but also vessels and objects of wood and of earthenware, and some are for honorable (noble, good) use and some for dishonorable (ignoble, common).*
>
> *Therefore, if anyone cleanses himself from these things [which are dishonorable—disobedient, sinful], he will be a vessel for honor, sanctified [set apart for a special purpose and], useful to the Master, prepared for every good work."*

I know from reading scripture that spiritual warfare is happening all around us. The last thing the enemy wants is for you to walk dressed in the identity God has given you. I also know the flesh (sinful nature) and the world (unrighteous culture) are at war against your potential.

You must level up as a Believer and take action in what you can control. God doesn't want you to be immature or lukewarm (Revelation 3:16). He wants Godly men and women who love Him and will learn, grow, and take responsibility in caring for His living temple. The Bible calls this stewardship.

<u>Don't miss this:</u> Not by satisfying your

desires, but by being good stewards

of what God has given you. Life.

It's an act of worship to honor and care for what God has created—body, mind, and spirit.

Romans 12:1 AMP, *"Therefore I urge you, brothers and sisters, by the mercies of God, to present your bodies [dedicating all of yourselves, set apart] as a living sacrifice, holy and well-pleasing to God, which is your rational (logical, intelligent) act of worship."*

1 Corinthians 3:1-3 AMP, *"However, brothers and sisters, I could not talk to you as to spiritual people, but [only] as to worldly people [dominated by human nature], mere infants [in the new life] in Christ! I fed you with milk, not solid food; for you were not yet able to receive it. Even now you are still not ready.*

> *You are still worldly [controlled by ordinary impulses, the sinful capacity]. For as long as there is jealousy and strife and discord among you, are you not unspiritual, and are you not walking like ordinary men [unchanged by faith]?"*

No longer should you, or can you, go on giving into the lusts of this world. Overindulging in social media and food, while sexualized fitness, easy access to drinking/drugs, "busyness," self-centeredness, and the stress of performance stand in your way. They pull you away from who you truly are called to be, what you were created for. *Greatness.*

Because of this, I believe it's necessary to learn to plan, prioritize, and build healthy habits for your entire being. Thus, taking intentional action in all areas of your life to stay consistent in your health and walk with God.

> Romans 8:10-11 AMP, *"If Christ lives in you, though your [natural] body is dead because of sin, your spirit is alive because of righteousness [which He provides]. And if the Spirit of Him who raised Jesus from the dead lives in you, He who raised Christ Jesus from the dead will also give life to your mortal bodies through His Spirit, who lives in you."*

As you are a balance of the physical and the spiritual, my philosophy is a balance of the practical and the biblical. The Holy Spirit, who quickens your own, is just as much a part of your wellness as the mind and body, actually allowing you the self-control and mind of Christ needed to walk consistently in this way of life (not by how much we strive to change).

> John 16:7 AMP, *"But I tell you the truth, it is your advantage that I go away; for if I do not go away, the helper (comforter, advocate, intercessor – counselor, strengthener, standby) will not come to you; but if I go, I will send Him (the Holy Spirit) to you [to be in close fellowship with you]."*

To put it plainly, you are changed from the inside out by your time spent with the Lord, His presence, and receiving it daily (2 Corinthians 3:17). I refer to this as "true rest," or what some call "devotional rest".

Yet, it can be one of the most difficult things to obtain with consistency. Damon Thompson, a worldwide revivalist, says it this way:

> *"The most difficult thing you'll say yes*
>
> *to in your life, is an end to personal,*
>
> *devotional inconsistency."*

This is where prioritizing organization, faith, and spiritual strength come in (we'll dive deeper into these ideas later in Chapter 7 – Body, Mind, and Spirit).

Finally, I present you with the keys of 360wellness that make up the foundation of my philosophy on wholeness: *Recovery, Exercise, Nutrition, Mindfulness, and Faith.*

In each chapter of this book, you will learn more about each individual key, and by exploring these five concepts through a biblical lens, I trust you can and will live a fulfilled life through every mountain and valley.

You will be prepared to love God and others with a content and purpose-driven heart, the way God intended for all of us.

Living with greatness.

<u>The 5 Whys:</u>

Before we begin, this coaching exercise will help smoothen your process. It will also help you identify and remember the deeper, personal meaning of this book and how it relates to you.

Take your time, answering each *why*, starting with your reason for reading *You Were Created For Greatness*. The following *whys* will begin to break down the true root of your purpose. May God bless you and guide you.

There is space to complete on the next page.

1. *Why are you reading this book?*

2. *Awesome. Why?*

3. *Ok, and why is this important to you?*

4. *Why?*

5. *Lastly, Why?*

Reflect

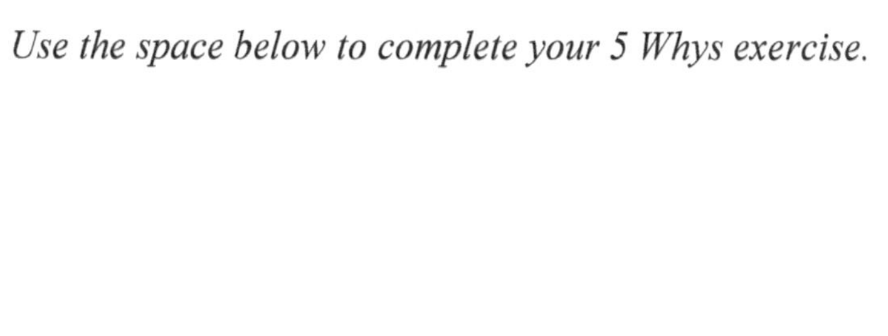

Use the space below to complete your 5 Whys exercise.

Thank you. This is your root, or core belief and

purpose behind choosing to read this book!

Chapter II – Recovery

*"The LORD is my Shepherd [to feed, to guide and to shield me], I shall
not want. He lets me lie down in green pastures; He leads me beside
the still and quiet waters. He refreshes and restores my soul (life); He
leads me in the paths of righteousness for His name's sake."*

Psalm 23:1-3 AMP

Ask yourself, *"Do I give enough to myself,*

to give my best to others?"

You must care for yourself to care well for others. This holds
true in all areas of life. You can't give what you don't have (for
long). So, if the answer is "no," this chapter is for you.

There's a fine line between powering through an injury or
burnout and humbling yourself to receive help. I've seen God use
these many times to teach and slow people down (including
myself).

Before I start with anyone looking to improve their
performance, health, fitness, diet, and/or lifestyle habits, I
encourage holistic *recovery* as a priority. It's fair to say nine out
of ten people currently deal with either pain, injury (current or
past), poor sleep, and stress in their body or mind that can create,
what I call, an imbalance. We all deal with things daily that pull
us away from being in a balanced state of wholeness.

In order to stay consistent in life and come from a place of abundance, you must build an internal, holistic balance from the inside out. To acknowledge this and then act on that awareness is foundational to your health.

Literally.

Please acknowledge this: you must *make time* to recover and balance yourself if you are going to stay consistent in your walk for the long haul. I find these benefits include, but are not limited to minimizing distractions, maximizing potential, enjoying the process, and preventing burnout wherever God calls you. Sometimes, you may just need to *rest*.

Particularly if you're reading this coming out of 2020, your body has been in a chronic state of stress and isolation, which can cause more than one health problem. In a world of striving and progress, we must learn to slow down and trust God within the storms.

Have you read Zechariah 4:6?

> *Then he said to me, "This is the word of the Lord to Zerubbabel, saying, 'Not by might nor by power, but by My Spirit,' says the Lord of armies."*

As humans, we tend to choose *striving* over *striding*. Yet, in addition to practical application, as a child of God you now have someone who fights on your behalf and can give you the strength you need in any weakness.

> 2 Corinthians 12:10 AMP, *"So I am well pleased with weaknesses, with insults, with distresses, with persecutions, and with difficulties, for the sake of Christ; for when I am weak [in human strength], then I am strong [truly able, truly powerful, truly drawing from God's strength]."*

The idea is to "abide."

This is the final piece: seeking God and His Word,

finding rest for your spirit—which adds rest

to your mind, body, and soul.

Now, through experience in my own life, along with a wide range of clients, I have found that whether you are active or sedentary, you must take the time to balance and recover yourself through intentional rest.

The human body is adaptive and smart, yet fragile. It can adjust to your workload, posture, hobbies, lifestyle, and daily habits but sooner or later imbalances begin to show. It is only a matter of time, usually in the form of burnout, including things such as pain, injury, anxiety, and/or "tightness" in the body (surprisingly, tightness has been found to be a neurological affect more than a tight "knot" in the muscle as people once believed).

Think of a car. The faster you go, the more pressure is put on the engine, shocks, and tires. If the car is not aligned (e.g., imbalances, low-tire pressure, dirty oil), you will experience wear and tear, not to mention low performance. In some cases, it may even begin to fall apart. However, *You Were Made to Move.*

This is one *360 Mindset* I have based 360wellness on. To take it one step further: *you were made to move, well!*

I want to see you progress and live a joyful, balanced, pain-free life, and it starts with a foundation of recovery. On the following pages I provide five practical ways to integrate more of it into your life today.

1. Relax, take a walk

Sometimes it can be simple. Taking the time to slow down for a five-minute walk has been shown to do wonders for stress management and boosting muscle recovery. Lowering stress levels can calm the nervous system (in turn lowering cortisol) and cause us to "reset" in the middle of the day, at the end of a stressful work-shift, or even as we get the day started off right.

Fun fact: the release of cortisol is a normal and helpful anti-inflammatory response. However, if released chronically, it can lead to health issues such as weight gain and increased inflammation. It can even negatively affect your immune system.

2. Targeted therapy

Many people don't know this, but 360wellness was founded on my creation of a physical therapy style: combining targeted massage with active stretching. The keyword here is *targeted*. By localizing the area of tension and pain, you can recover the body faster, adding efficiency to your recovery routine.

If possible, especially when dealing with pain or injury, search for a therapist in your area who focuses on acute, therapeutic massage.

It's ok, you can take care of yourself!

Not into massage? Is it not in your budget? No worries, I can relate. So, I bring you another option and a great tool (not a solution)—foam rollers. A foam roller releases muscle tension by improving blood flow.

You can lay on it, press against the wall, or use it in a seated chair position. This release is temporary, as the body will usually go back to its "comfortable" position (posture is commonly formed through repetitive movements and mood), but it's a great start and has become a part of many athletes' recovery routine.

3. Breathe deep

Just five deep breaths a day can be a great start in reducing stress, lowering your heart rate and blood pressure, all while decreasing your cortisol levels. I recommend setting a timer on your phone when you know your day is at its busiest to remind yourself and help break the cycle of stress. You can take this small, daily action and put it to use for a surprising boost to your wellness.

Try this: "Box Breathing" is an awesome tool to slow down, breathe deep, and maximize your oxygen intake. Start by inhaling for five seconds (through your nose), then hold for five seconds, exhale for five seconds (through your mouth), and hold at the bottom for five seconds; then repeat. It takes a little bit of getting used to, but only one round may be just what you need to reset during a stressful day.

4. Movement is medicine

Not many people think of movement itself as recovery. I am thankful for many great mentors in my life, showing me the way. One of them, Dominick Nusdeu of Motion Mechanix showed me the value of movement as a substitute to massage therapy.

Yes, replacing massage with movement. As I was a licensed massage therapist, we had our brotherly disagreements, but he pointed me to a view of how the body functions that I hadn't seen before. His concept was to create stability, or strength in certain ranges of motion. This is meant to challenge your mobility and find strength in an array of different movements (what he calls "configurations").

The basic principle is this: you must stabilize the specific joint associated with pain/tightness with movement.

When these range of motion exercises are applied over time, most tightness, pain, and lack of stability in the joints disappear.

If your shoulder is experiencing tightness, stabilize it. If your knee is experiencing pain, stabilize it. And so on. Time and time again, I've seen pain, tension, and "tightness" all be caused by instability of the joint (which happens to also affect your posture and strength). If you start with small movements to improve the posture and connection of the focused area, the relief will amaze you. I could write all day about this, but I'll leave you with one last tip:

If you move a certain direction, and there is pain/discomfort, stop and try the same movement but in the opposite direction (and hold).

So, for example, if your knee bothers you when bending, straighten it out and hold for five to seconds (like a knee extension exercise). If your low back hurts when bending over, lay down and extend your hips with a bridge exercise. If your neck feels tight or has pain when turning to the left, slowly turn to the right and hold. This technique will begin to stabilize (or balance) the body's "push/pull" relationship.

Whether you are new to exercise or a seasoned expert, you can begin to apply this technique today for a great start to recovery. To help, here's what it could look like if you organized these into your warm-up routine:

1. *Seated Knee Extensions*
   2 sets of 3 reps (5 second hold)

2. *Bridges*
   2 sets of 3 reps (5 second hold)

3. *Neck Rotations*
   2 sets of 3 reps (5 second hold)

5. Sleep is king

Maybe the MOST important factor of physical and mental recovery is sleep. Research has shown sleep is the most powerful recovery technique you can give to yourself, and it's free! Praise the Lord.

Between *seven and nine* hours is considered a healthy range. However, just as important of a factor is sleep *quality*. This is a personal goal of mine (something that I must stay mindful of daily) and another *360 Mindset* I live by: *Quality Over Quantity.* You can sleep for hours, but if it's not quality, deep sleep, you will not get the full RECOVERY benefits.

So, here are a few restful ideas to implement into your growing holistic lifestyle, thanks to **Precision Nutrition**, a world-renowned nutrition and lifestyle-coaching program.

While just a few ideas are provided, I encourage you to highlight those that relate to you. Then choose *ONE* to focus on and apply for one to two weeks until you have built a new habit.

Here are my top six ideas:

- <u>Stick to a routine bedtime</u>
    - the mind and body like consistent timing

- <u>Turn off electronics at least thirty minutes before bed</u>
    - screen time can reduce your sleep quality (melatonin)

- <u>Journal</u>
    - write out your thoughts, ideas, and/or emotions to help ease your mind

- <u>Keep your room dark</u>
    - add blackout curtains or try a sleep mask to promote deep, "REM" sleep

- <u>Exercise regularly</u>
  - aim for twenty to sixty minutes daily. This promotes restful sleep and helps manage your energy

- Apply five-minutes of prayer to your bed-time routine
  - spend time with God and rest in the "secret place" of His presence.

Psalm 91 (NIV) is one of my favorite passages to read out loud and *rest* (meditate) in before bed. This is a song of King David who had a deep, personal relationship with God. Don't worry, we'll dive deeper into this specific kind of "rest" in Chapter 7.

¹ Whoever dwells in the shelter of the Most High
will rest in the shadow of the Almighty.

² I will say of the LORD, "He is my refuge and my fortress,
my God, in whom I trust."

³ Surely he will save you
from the fowler's snare
and from the deadly pestilence.

⁴ He will cover you with his feathers,
and under his wings you will find refuge;
His faithfulness will be your shield and rampart.

⁵ You will not fear the terror of night,
nor the arrow that flies by day,

⁶ nor the pestilence that stalks in the darkness,
nor the plague that destroys at midday.

7 A thousand may fall at your side,
ten thousand at your right hand,
but it will not come near you.

8 You will only observe with your eyes
and see the punishment of the wicked.

9 If you say, "The LORD is my refuge,"
and you make the Most High your dwelling,

10 no harm will overtake you,
no disaster will come near your tent.

11 For he will command his angels concerning you
to guard you in all your ways;

12 they will lift you up in their hands,
so that you will not strike your foot against a stone.

13 You will tread on the lion and the cobra;
you will trample the great lion and the serpent.

14 "Because he loves me," says the LORD, "I will rescue him;
I will protect him, for he acknowledges my name.

15 He will call on me, and I will answer him;
I will be with him in trouble,
I will deliver him and honor him.

16 With long life I will satisfy him
and show him my salvation."

In the next chapter, we will dive into my concept of exercise and how you can use simple actions to help improve your life for the better.

Yet first, as Believers, we must differentiate the Church and our mentality from the way the world sees fitness and health.

Reflect

Think back to this question: Do I give enough to myself to give my best to others?

Consider the 5 practical ways to integrate recovery into your life. What do you want to start incorporating this week?

What is one small action you can take to accomplish this?

Chapter III – Exercise

"And do not be conformed to this world [any longer with its superficial values and customs], but be transformed and progressively changed [as you mature spiritually] by the renewing of your mind, so that you may prove [for yourselves] what the will of God is, that which is good and acceptable and perfect [in His plan and purpose for you]."

Romans 12:2 AMP

Growing up, exercise was simple. For me as a kid, it involved tag, hide and go seek, dodgeball, you name it. It was easy, and it was fun. There were no strings attached, and there was no real pressure to look or be a certain way.

As we grow up, however, the idea of exercise begins to take a shift. Things change. Unfortunately, most of what movies, commercials, personal trainers, social media, and gyms promote is a "sexualized" kind of fitness.

This way of living is not sustainable or healthy for many reasons. Many of you are tempted to aim for unrealistic goals, setting you up for lies and disappointment. Instead, let us focus on this: God loves you no matter your size, shape, or how "different" you may feel.

There is a deeper meaning and purpose

to life than to satisfy the physical need

or image the world reflects.

Everyone else may be doing it, even striving for it, yet you are called to stand out from the crowd and not give in. You are called to go so far as to continually transform your mind, leading as new examples to others *counterintuitive* to the ways of this world.

It is important for us as the Church to understand that exercise focused solely on our image will not produce the good fruit or freedom we desire. As small as it may be, the enemy can use this foothold in your life to plant lies and distract you from your true identity. This understanding is especially essential as the fitness industry only continues to expand and sexualize this kind of image-based fitness.

So, I call you back to the basics. Exercise, no matter what it looks like, is important for a healthy life. Let's review the definition.

According to Oxford Dictionary, exercise is *"a process or activity carried out for a specific purpose, especially one concerned with a specified area or skill."*

I love this definition because no matter the specifics, *you* are taking action for a *purpose.* Some may define this as being intentional. Consistent health is all about intention, and I genuinely believe you were made for an active life! The body is capable of more than you challenge it with, so I encourage you to have fun and explore that potential. Along with this, there are hundreds of benefits to exercise.

Here are just a few that stand out to me:

1. Improves circulation
2. Increases bone density
3. Can prevent depression/anxiety
4. Challenges your comfort-zone (boosts mental toughness)
5. Supports daily energy and quality sleep

The more you stay moving, the better chance you have at living a robust, happy, long, and healthy life. With factors ranging from stress-relief, weight control, and pain management, I have seen movement improve quality of life from the young to the old.

360 Mindset:

"Movement is Medicine."

Through my work with many clients dealing with pain, I have seen the healing benefits of movement. Again, it may seem counterintuitive, but staying active is the one thing that outshines other passive rehabilitation and prevention techniques. It is effective and free. All you must do is start moving, with *intention*.

Think of a child in development: moldable, eager, and willing to try new things. No matter what type of exercise you prefer, I encourage you to keep this simplicity at heart and stick to the basics.

Remember, *"physical training is of some value"* so let us apply it with purity in our lives; a little can go a long way, allowing you to focus on the more valuable areas in your life without getting carried away (more on these in Chapter 6 - Faith).

"Ok," you may ask, "but what does this look like?"

Here are a few examples I would share with my personal clients:

1. Organize a walking routine

Whether indoor, on a hiking trail, or in your neighborhood set a day and time in your weekly schedule. Start small with five-minutes and watch a new habit evolve.

It's all about building a consistent routine as a building block to your wellness. You can get creative: short on time? Combine your goals and use walking as a devotional time between you and God. He deserves it and longs to fellowship with you daily.

2. Join a team sport

Soccer leagues, softball, tennis, basketball, volleyball— the options are endless. Building a community around your activity helps with consistency and support in the long run!

You were built for community.

3. Add an active hobby

Pick up a new hobby like bike riding, hiking, swimming, golf, or kickboxing as a great way to stay moving. The more you are outdoors and breathing in fresh air the better. This can help melt away stress and allow you to "be in the moment."

4. Movement Therapy™

This is a term I have coined and implemented into my sessions with clients. It can be a form of intentional "yoga," rehab, corrective exercise, or active stretching which can lead you to preventing pain and injury while improving your mobility.

Movement Therapy includes specific, customized movements to help slow things down and move your body in new ways, releasing tension and stress, while activating key muscles. It could be as simple as building a small active-stretching routine you can apply daily to your life.

If you feel good in this area, feel free to skip to the next point, but here are a few movements that promote healthy mobility:

<u>Straight Leg Raises:</u> this is great for releasing the hamstrings, activating the core, and protecting the lower back. Start on your back with both knees bent. You will then straighten one leg out, lift it up to your maximum range of motion, then lower down to the floor.

Repeat for a few reps, about ten, and then switch. During this movement, focus on your breath and keep the working leg straight to activate your quad (thigh) and core, in turn allowing your hamstrings to relax. Ten reps of two sets each leg would be a great start. If you are experiencing low back pain, couple this with the bridge exercise.

<u>Seated Trunk Rotation + Extension:</u> this is great for your mid-back, shoulders, and neck. Start in a seated chair position and practice rotating to your left and right (as far as you can) with your arms crossed over your chest. Stay mindful of your breathing. Once you reach your full turn to one side, slowly stretch down (as if crunching), and then while staying turned, activate your back by extending upward back to sitting position.

Repeat on both sides for a few reps. Five reps of two sets each side would be a great start. *Retest each side at the end to see if you've improved your mobility!*

<u>Seated Trunk Side Bend:</u> this is one of my favorites and great for those with lower or mid-back pain. You will start in a seated chair position. Cross your arms over your chest and then slowly breathe out while crunching to the side away from your pain a few times (to both sides if there's no pain).

Make sure to stay mindful and move slow. Just five reps of two sets can yield beneficial results.

5. Build a resistance training routine

Weighted exercise comes with many benefits such as improved bone density, mood, and muscle mass. As you age, bone density and muscle mass become more valuable for long life and vitality. Resistance training is the gold standard but choose what you enjoy.

Remember everyone is different, you don't have to do what others do or sign up for a gym membership to get active. I personally enjoy body weight exercises, resistance bands, and free weights— such as kettlebells.

Here is an example of a circuit training routine I would create for efficiency and preventing injury to use with my clients. It encompasses a full body approach, while staying mindful of posture and balancing exercises to promote mobility and well-being (not just another "killer" workout).

If you don't know the exercise, use your friendly search engine such as Google to help.

I call it Corrective Circuit Training™

1. *Resistance Band Row - twelve reps*
2. *Weighted Goblet Squat - twelve reps*
3. *Plank Hold - thirty seconds*
4. *Air Squats - thirty reps*

Aim to complete four rounds, with minimal rest. Challenge yourself, get creative, and have fun in fifteen minutes or less! If you try this workout, post about it on Instagram and tag me @360wellness for a feature. #YWCFG

And so, I encourage you to explore something new from these five examples above and write down a few ways you can apply it to your life, today. Every day is a new day. You have so much to enjoy and be thankful for, including the freedom to move.

This calls for *gratitude*.

From God alone, you are given another day to

breathe, move, and enjoy life with others.

You must stay reminded of the humility in all of this. Thankfulness for another day goes a long way, and taking a walk to remember your purpose sure beats stressing out about your image or the thoughts of others. *Don't forget, when you take care of the inside, the outside will reflect.*

Today's culture is begging for you to give into self-consciousness and ego. Don't believe the lies. You must step away from these negative thoughts and receive God's love for yourself daily. He is what matters most. Not our six-pack, the amount of likes we get on social media, or even who we date or marry will ever outweigh this truth of His abundant love.

Romans 8:38-39 AMP, *"For I am convinced [and continue to be convinced—beyond any doubt] that neither death, nor life, nor angels, nor principalities, nor things present and threatening, nor things to come, nor powers, nor height, nor depth, nor any other created thing, will be able to separate us from the [unlimited] love of God, which is in Christ Jesus our Lord."*

In turn, through honoring your body, caring for it to promote health and well-being, you can reverse and prevent many forms of pain, sickness, and disease. Not to mention, you can live a happier and more capable life for God and others.

I'm convinced that in most of the world today, with all the "luxury" (compared to third-world countries) and limited activity in our jobs or school, you must constantly be proactive with your health, and for the right reasons. You have an opportunity today to respond, not merely listen. In the United States and around the world, a sedentary lifestyle will only become more common as technology increases.

If you don't build healthy exercise habits now, you may pay the bigger price later. No longer can you rely on your jobs or daily to-do list to ensure strength and longevity as your ancestors once did. Believers must be examples of endurance and discipline in every area of our life. This is "mind over matter. And matter over mind." How you handle and challenge your physical self affects your mind/spirit, and vice versa.

> 2 Timothy 1:7 AMP, *"For God did not give us a spirit of timidity or cowardice or fear, but [He has given us a spirit] of power and of love and of sound judgment and personal discipline [abilities that result in a calm, well-balanced mind and self-control]."*

Lastly, the concept of mental toughness has been on my heart. The art of exercise can be used as a tool to build mental strength and self-discipline. There is truth to this, and as the world indulges in "easy," it would be wise to challenge your comfort zone and resist the temptation of laziness, even "sloth."

> Proverbs 6:9 AMP, *"How long will you lie down, O lazy one? When will you arise from your sleep [and learn self-discipline]?"*

There's a saying that goes, "If you're not growing, you're dying." As a Believer you must challenge your body, mind, and spirit to ensure growth to be at your best; to feel alive!

Discomfort is what

builds greatness.

You don't grow by being comfortable, and you don't get a diamond without a little pressure. Whatever way you want to look at it, step back and consider how you can apply exercise to start challenging your comfort zone today. This may feel like just "more work" at first, but trust me, it will only build you up and make you stronger in the long run.

Christians should be some of the healthiest people on earth, setting an example of wellness for the world. Imagine if you walked out your life with active intention, challenging yourself daily in all areas of life, while staying strong (physically and mentally) to love and impact the lives of others around you.

Can you imagine yourself now?

Take a moment. What would that look like to you? What if you lived to be a giver and a solid foundation to those in need, even into old age? Exercise may attribute to a small portion in this equation, but it's still a portion. Do not neglect your body. You are only given one.

I don't know who this is for but it's hard and I understand. Life gets thrown at you, yet don't let the excuse of denying the flesh empower yourself to neglect God's temple (yourself).

There is a difference between caring for the body God has given you and denying yourself. It may be a thin line, but you must acknowledge this: no longer can we as a Church continue allowing pain, injury, sickness, and the like to occur just because we were not good stewards of our own body. Sometimes it's not spiritual warfare, it's just you. We are all capable of becoming our worst enemy at times.

So, I challenge you now. Utilize your time today, start your new season, and continue moving forward to grow into the full potential God has given you. It could start with a simple practice such as planning and "making the time" for that five-minute workout, organizing your health as a priority, or going the extra mile to care for someone in need (even when you're busy).

In the next chapter, you will discover just how you can gain greater control over your lifestyle, continue to prevent health issues, and make conscious, mindful, self-controlled choices to be at your best. And it starts with the power of *nutrition*.

Reflect

How would your life change if you began to challenge yourself with intentional exercise?

How could you begin to lay an active, healthy foundation for your new lifestyle TODAY?

If you lived to be 100 years old, what would you want to be known for?

Chapter IV – Nutrition

1 Peter 5:8 AMP, *"Be sober [well balanced and self-disciplined], be alert and cautious at all times. That enemy of yours, the devil, prowls around like a roaring lion [fiercely hungry], seeking someone to devour."*

Nutrition is your foundation. From your physical, mental, to spiritual self, sound nutrition stands strong as a leader in health and transformation. Let me explain.

If you think about eating and satisfying the body (flesh), they go hand in hand. It is our most basic and primitive action. What you consume and why you consume it matters.

Yet, it's often the one thing Believers, pastors, and missionaries "let go" or overlook. I've seen it time and time again, even experiencing it myself— especially on mission trips. We tend to be comfortable with "getting everything else right" while letting our diet suffer because we "deserve it" or we think, "what's the harm" (when there's grace)?

I believe we are missing a powerful *opportunity* here.

Many of us know the power of fasting in our prayer life and the positive effect it has in our walk as Believers. After fasting from food, however, we tend to go back to living as we did before. It's normal. Yet, it's this inconsistent way of life I challenge you on.

What if you practiced setting aside your desires and denied certain eating and drinking habits that hindered your spiritual, mental, and physical potential, consistently?

In doing this, I believe the holistic benefits of "fasting" could be experienced more continual and long-term. Or maybe you have never practiced fasting before. Wherever you are at, I would like to introduce a new thought.

When you slow down and set your focus on healthy

nutrition as a priority, your life will change.

Whether you are a student, business executive, working mom, pastor, missionary, nutrition expert, or a combination, healthy habits go a long way in promoting not only the vitality of your body and mind, but also your spirit.

One could say, "spiritual clarity?"

I think of healthy eating primarily as *self-control and self-care*. Applying these as spiritual practices to your diet feeds into your daily lifestyle, as well as your relationship with God (no pun intended). It's not that fasting, or self-denial brings us any closer to God, but that we clear away the distractions or "static" of the flesh. For the flesh and the Spirit are in opposition.

> Galatians 5:17 AMP, *"For the sinful nature has its desire which is opposed to the Spirit, and the [desire of the] Spirit opposes the sinful nature; for these [two, the sinful nature and the Spirit] are in direct opposition to each other [continually in conflict], so that you [as believers] do not [always] do whatever [good things] you want to do."*

When you are constantly feeding (literally) every want and need of the flesh, it can seep into other areas of your life. Sin always starts subtle. We must stay "alert and cautious" (1 Peter 5:8) to live a life of purity and consistency for the Kingdom.

Christ was sent to restore your spirit, why squander it?

> Romans 8:3-4 AMP, *"For what the Law could not do [that is, overcome sin and remove its penalty, its power] being weakened by the flesh [man's nature without the Holy Spirit], God did: He sent His own Son in the likeness of sinful man as an offering for sin.*
>
> *And He condemned sin in the flesh [subdued it and overcame it in the person of His own Son], so that the [righteous and just] requirement of the Law might be fulfilled in us who do not live our lives in the ways of the flesh [guided by worldliness and our sinful nature], but [live our lives] in the ways of the Spirit [guided by His power]."*

Please hang with me here. Practically, for example, sugar or similar "ultra-flavor foods" (e.g., salty/savory) are known to be "addictive," almost "irresistible" by design—or at the very least can have an influence on your behavior (through dopamine, serotonin, and the like).

A small amount of influence goes farther than you think. And regardless of choice, this influence (or effect) changes the way you think, and therefore act.

Back in 2016, during a time I had in prayer with God, I came to a revelation while I myself was struggling with eating habits along with on and off depression.

"If everything is a choice, including loving God,

then eating foods that hinder our choices

probably isn't a good idea."

Read that one more time.

Love is a choice. The scriptures have always called you to *action*. There is grace, but God wants you to step out in faith. Even when you try your best (which will never be enough) the Lord's grace catches you, filling in what you never could because He loves you. This is relationship. This is unconditional love.

> Matthew 22:37 AMP, *"And Jesus replied to him, 'You shall love the Lord your God with all your heart, and with all your soul, and with all your mind.'"*

> 1 Corinthians 8:3AMP, *"But if anyone loves God [with awe-filled reverence, obedience and gratitude], he is known by Him [as His very own and is greatly loved]."*

> 1 John 4:21 AMP, *"And this commandment we have from Him, that the one who loves God should also [unselfishly] love his brother and seek the best for him."*

> 1 John 5:2 AMP, *"By this we know [without any doubt] that we love the children of God: [expressing that love] when we love God and obey His commandments."*

All these scriptures state love as a verb.

Now, to continue my story. As I was working as a personal trainer and sports massage therapist, I became surprised when I saw how food could impact everyday behavior. Although I was just beginning my journey into business and my relationship with God was deepening, I had continued revelations that branched off this "sugar" topic.

As mentioned earlier I was going through up and down depression, along with seasons of poor food and lifestyle choices. I just wasn't thinking straight or consistently. I knew this wasn't me, and it wasn't from God. As we know from scripture, we can battle against spiritual warfare (demonic forces), our flesh (natural desires), and the world (sinful culture). This was one of those times I could feel it was a combination. My flesh was getting in the way, and I felt the enemy was using it against me while I was genuinely seeking God.

There are many tactics the enemy can use against you that rarely seem "demonic," but you must not forget the devil is subtle and crafty. If he can't beat you, he sure can try to confuse and attack your mind. This is one reason why I am so passionate about nutrition. I see a lot of the mental battles people go through today actually being caused from a poor diet and lifestyle, yet we call them "mental health issues" and get prescribed medication or try to self sooth with more toxic habits (such as excess alcohol, drugs, even pornography).

This is not the way.

And so, from that point forward, I felt led to go on a fast. Not just any fast, but one that removed common indulging and satisfying food and drink. From my scientific background, you could say all things that released high levels of "dopamine."

What is *dopamine*?

A quote from <u>Into Action Recovery Center</u> describes dopamine as, *"one of the 'feel good' chemicals in our brain. Interacting with the pleasure and reward center of our brain, dopamine — along with other chemicals like serotonin, oxytocin, and endorphins — plays a vital role in how happy we feel. In addition to our mood, dopamine also affects movement, memory, and focus. Healthy levels of dopamine drive us to seek and repeat pleasurable activities, while low levels can have an adverse physical and psychological impact."*

They go on to say, *"imbalances in these chemicals impact our behavior and quality of life and can create a vast amount of health issues,"* including a list below:

- Anxiety
- Addiction
- Behavioral disturbances
- Cognitive disorders
- Diseases (Such as Parkinson's)
- Fatigue
- Hormonal imbalances
- Mood disorders
- Obesity
- Pain

This is where science and faith meet. Isn't God good?

Some things in the Bible that feel like they "limit" our lifestyle or happiness may actually be meant for our own good, whether we realize it or not. After doing my research, I began making a list of everything that can influence you in this way to an unhealthy degree.

I came up with these seven:

- Added Sugar
- Smoking/Drugs
- Social Media
- Highly Processed Foods
- Caffeine
- Sexual Activity
- Alcohol

These seven stood out to me as the most common and influential factors we deal with today. Then one week after I wrote about these things in my notebook, something happened. While I was in prayer, I heard the Lord speak to my heart (I always describe receiving a word from God as an "overriding thought").

"I want you to fast of these things,

until Sunday the 19th."

(Key word Sunday)

I reacted thinking, "Pshh, last week was the 19th. This wasn't from God."

Yeah, last week was the 19th. And it seemed God wanted me to fast from these things for three full weeks. I checked the calendar, and sure enough the 19th of the following month fell on a Sunday (it happened to be exactly twenty-one days) to solidify my belief.

Crazy? Well, God knows your heart and can speak to it. Sometimes you just have to be still; and *listen*.

I have concluded that whenever there is an important shift or transition in my life or around it, God encourages me to fast. It may be for unseen reasons, but I also know from experience it heightens my sensitivity to Him, limiting the flesh that can get in the way. His ways are always higher than mine.

> Isaiah 55:8-9 AMP, *" 'For My thoughts are not your thoughts, Nor are your ways My ways,' declares the Lord. 'For as the heavens are higher than the earth, So are My ways higher than your ways And My thoughts higher than your thoughts.'"*

<u>The bottom line:</u>

Fasting cleanses your body, mind, and

spirit by limiting the flesh and

empowering the Spirit.

I always sense and hear God more clearly during a fast and have heard the same from others. And so, there I was. This basically left me with water, whole foods, and the Bible (I don't recommend eating your Bible).

Believe me, the first few days were not easy (and I mean not easy), but after that, something opened up. It's amazing the control these factors can have over our life, yet rarely do we realize it.

During my fast, I experienced an increase in clarity, focus, energy, motivation, and self-control. I had never felt better! God was showing me the powerful effects a healthy diet and lifestyle could have on my life and in turn those around me.

He wants us to shine bright. And so, I want to share this secret with you. I call it the ***21-Day: Dopamine Reset***. As mentioned above, you will cut out these pleasurable foods, drinks, and/or habits for twenty-one days (get ready for the fun!).

Trust me, you will not regret it. This can be used as an annual reset for your body, mind, and spirit or as a consistent lifestyle change you create to thrive in the Spirit and in life—whatever it throws at you.

The official list is as follows:

1. Added Sugar (all kinds, e.g., honey, white, organic)
2. Smoking/Drugs (cigarettes, marijuana, etc.)
3. Social Media (Facebook, Instagram, Twitter, etc.)
4. Processed Foods (bread, cheese, chips, etc.)
5. Caffeine (coffee, green tea, etc.)
6. Sexual Activity
7. Alcohol

If you feel that cutting out all that have influence in your life at once is too much to handle, I understand. I recommend you make a swift change for best results but choosing one area to focus on and building from there works as well.

I like to say, there's no point in a perfect program if no one is doing it. In that case, I would encourage you to start with the easiest choice and work toward your most challenging until all that apply are denied. This will allow you to build momentum and healthy habits that hopefully will last once the twenty-one days are over.

You may not deal with all seven of these areas, so if one doesn't apply to you, great! No matter the number of factors you choose, work toward twenty-one days and let yourself reset and rest from all that the world indulges in.

Your body, mind, and spirit will thank you and I believe God will reward your faithfulness in this season. *Abide in Him during this time, and you will not fail.*

Yes, it will not be easy, and the flesh is weak, but if this fast feels like the right choice for you, I encourage you to *pray*. Ask God for the strength and grace needed during this time. You must remember in your weakness, He is strong, and it's not by your own strength but by His Spirit.

> Zechariah 4:6 AMP, *"Then he said to me, "This [continuous supply of oil] is the word of the Lord to Zerubbabel [prince of Judah], saying, 'Not by might, nor by power, but by My Spirit [of whom the oil is a symbol],' says the Lord of hosts."*

> 2 Corinthians 12:10 AMP, *"So I am well pleased with weaknesses, with insults, with distresses, with persecutions, and with difficulties, for the sake of Christ; for when I am weak [in human strength], then I am strong [truly able, truly powerful, truly drawing from God's strength]."*

The main purpose of this fast is to help you reset and take back control of your thoughts, actions, and emotions that may have been affected by poor nutrition, social media, and other behaviors. This is different from your average fast in which you abstain from food for a few days. This practice is meant to integrate into your daily life, boosting your self-control and discipline while giving to God as an act of worship (by denying the flesh).

Romans 12:1 AMP, *"Therefore I urge you, brothers and sisters, by the mercies of God, to present your bodies [dedicating all of yourselves, set apart] as a living sacrifice, holy and well-pleasing to God, which is your rational (logical, intelligent) act of worship."*

This is where the body, mind, and spirit intersect,

as one truly affects the other.

From there, you can more easily transition into a consistently healthy lifestyle with fewer cravings, choosing to manage your diet the way you want, thus maximizing your health for the long run. You will also experience greater energy and focus and have a more positive outlook on life! If you are looking for more support or direction on this practice, please visit:

https://linktr.ee/360wellness

There's one last factor I would like to discuss specifically. *Caffeine*. Coffee is one of the leading drinks in this world that keeps us going. "It keeps the world turning," you might say.

Yet, throughout my personal experience of the **21-Day Reset**, I was surprised by how much I relied on coffee for energy. In the morning, in the afternoon, it was part of my daily routine. When I cut it out, I began withdrawals as an addict would experience when removing their drug of choice.

Headaches, depression, lack of motivation, mental fog, irritation, and the like all followed as I cut caffeine out of my life. Is this the way it's supposed to be?

I challenge your thinking today. Does caffeine have some benefits? Of course. I see it as a tool. Yet, as I walked into day four, day five, day six of the fast I realized that *food*, yes food, was my supplier of energy. I had to eat four to five medium-sized meals to keep up with my activity and work demands without caffeine. And do you know what?

I felt unstoppable. No longer was I slave to a substance I idolized for so long. The Lord gave you the sweet blessing of food and He has not called you to be slave to any man or thing. Yet, I see so many of us captured (or even addicted) by this simple ingredient.

> Romans 6:15-18 AMP, *"What then [are we to conclude]? Shall we sin because we are not under Law, but under [God's] grace? Certainly not!*
>
> *Do you not know that when you continually offer yourselves to someone to do his will, you are the slaves of the one whom you obey, either [slaves] of sin, which leads to death, or of obedience, which leads to righteousness (right standing with God)?*
>
> *But thank God that though you were slaves of sin, you became obedient with all your heart to the standard of teaching in which you were instructed and to which you were committed. And having been set free from sin, you have become the slaves of righteousness [of conformity to God's will and purpose]."*

So, I call you out of that place. As a child of God, I call you to overcome even the little things holding you back from fully walking in complete sonship to the Father. He is our Rock. He is our Source. Let us never forget this and be distracted by the lusts of this world that seem so innocent. For even Satan masquerades as an angel of light (2 Corinthians 11:14).

Give the enemy no foothold, for you are called to

walk with power, discipline, and authority by grace,

constantly attaining the mind of Christ and having

God first and foremost in your life.

This revelation sums up my thoughts on the power of food and the effects it can have on us. Am I perfect with all of this? Believe me, I am not. If someone brings in some donuts, sign me up! However, when I overindulge and give way to the flesh and its desires, I know ultimately the effect it can have on me. I have seen the other side.

When I slow down, reframe, and look ahead toward my long-term goals, I can often break the temptations that only lead to short-term satisfaction. Over time, it gets easier and easier. When you stay consistent, a kind of resilience builds up. Just like when you exercise, your muscles initially break down, yet you come back stronger. The same is true for your mind.

Now, let me be clear, I'm not saying processed foods, sugar, alcohol, and the like are "bad." I believe in balance, moderation, and a healthy relationship with these.

However, I also think it's important to be aware of your intentions, checking your heart, and knowing the negative side effects of these choices, which are so readily available in today's indulgent culture. There is no such thing as a "bad" food and food does not defile you. It's your "why", or heart that matters.

> Mark 7:15 AMP, *"there is nothing outside a man [such as food] which by going into him can defile him [morally or spiritually]; but the things which come out of [the heart of] a man are what defile and dishonor him."*

I know there is talk about distrust of the food and drink industry (or the social media), and how it can seem to be against us, causing sickness, obesity, depression, and anxiety.

We like to play the blame game, and this may be true in some instances. Maybe certain leaders in the industries are all about making money and marketing products regardless of the impact on our physical and mental health. But from personal experience, and what I believe God has shown me, I challenge you to look at things a little differently. YOU. Yes, you, are ultimately in control. My goal is to give you back the power.

I encourage you to hold every thought and action captive in your life. If you have to delete social media, then delete it. If you need to keep junk food out of your kitchen, then do it.

There's a saying from Precision Nutrition co-founder and CEO, John Berardi, which goes something like this, "If a food is in your house or possession, either you, someone you love, or someone you marginally tolerate will eventually eat it."

This is just human psychology. And what does Jesus say about temptation?

> Matthew 5:30 AMP, *"If your right hand makes you stumble and leads you to sin, cut it off and throw it away [that is, remove yourself from the source of temptation]; for it is better for you to lose one of the parts of your body than for your whole body to go into hell."*

Again, the flesh is weak, but the spirit is willing. God is stronger. This may be a fluid process with highs and lows, but I believe in you. Continually keep moving forward and let the grace of God daily into your life to attain the mind of Christ in all you do.

Amen.

> Matthew 26:41 AMP, *"Keep actively watching and praying that you may not come into temptation; the spirit is willing, but the body is weak."*

> *1* Corinthians 2:16 AMP, *"For WHO HAS KNOWN THE MIND and PURPOSES OF THE LORD, SO AS TO INSTRUCT HIM? But we have the mind of Christ [to be guided by His thoughts and purposes]."*

For example, can you see Jesus going to a party and indulging in all the chips? Probably not. Can you see Jesus struggling with His Starbucks or Instagram addiction? It's a bit funny to even think about. I don't think so.

He was fully centered in who

He was and although tempted as we are,

did not give into the lust of this world.

The enemy is subtle, and every sinful habit starts small. As Damon Thompson, a worldwide revivalist calls it, "one lamb at a time." This quote is based on the shepherds stewarding their flock and how we are to take every lamb, or in this case, thought and action into account. Because before you know it, your whole flock could be gone. So, don't give in to the little things, and you can prevent the greater.

You may say, "But my work is so stressful and busy. I don't have time to eat healthy!" That's fair. I understand there is a need for work and responsibilities take a priority; but is that really worth your mental health or the potential of a *greater* relationship with God and even others? Jesus says it Himself in Mark 8:36 (AMP).

"For what does it benefit a man to gain the whole world

[with all its pleasures], and forfeit his soul?"

This is just food for thought (geez really with the puns). I do not mean to overload you, but there is truly power in sound nutrition. All you have to do is start making small adjustments to your health, and I promise you, it doesn't take as much energy or time as you think. In fact, I believe it will give you more.

I heard a saying the other day that goes something like this,

"Most people spend their health seeking

wealth, to then only end up spending

their wealth seeking health."

Health truly is wealth. When you believe and walk out on these truths, you empower yourself through Christ to rise above the world's mentality. No longer are you walking in the way of the world, but you have taken the narrow path.

> Matthew 7:13-14 AMP, *"Enter through the narrow gate. For wide is the gate and broad and easy to travel is the path that leads the way to destruction and eternal loss, and there are many who enter through it. But small is the gate and narrow and difficult to travel is the path that leads the way to [everlasting] life, and there are few who find it."*

It can be lonely at times and against the grain, but it produces life for the present and the life to come (1 Timothy 4:8). You may say, "But it's everywhere! I feel like it is inevitable." Or, "I grew up with it. It's just a part of my culture."

Welcome to Jesus culture. Take every thought captive, beloved. If you are serious about change, then setting goals, setting plans, setting small daily actions, and setting up your environment for success are your keys to move against the grain of worldly influence with consistency.

Here are five prompts to help you write it out, putting pen to paper, and thoughts to action.

1. Mindset

> What can you set your mind on today? *Through Christ you have the fruit of the Spirit: love, joy, peace, patience, kindness, goodness, faithfulness, gentleness, and self-control* (Galatians 5:22-23). In the Spirit, you attain these.

So, on all occasions remind yourself of these truths; write them out, pray them over yourself, even when you don't "feel like it." Emotions come and go, but God is truth, and this is about conquering the flesh.

Remember, our identity is in Jesus. Always.

2. Goal

What does healthy eating or a healthy lifestyle look like to you? What do you want to improve but haven't in your life? For example, this could be anywhere from losing twenty pounds, to improving your mental health, to spending time with Jesus daily.

Now be specific. The further you can break down this goal to fit within your deeper "why" the better. For example: from I want to lose ten pounds, to I want to feel more athletic or live a long, healthy life.

Think, "what will result in my life when I accomplish my goal?" This is more subjective versus simply objective, which is often uncontrollable.

3. Plan

How are you going to do it? What skills or practices do you need to accomplish your bigger goal? For example, you want to start cooking at home.

A *practice* could be weekly grocery shopping, organizing your kitchen for success, or researching fresh recipes. Think about it. Get creative!

4. Small actions

Now break those practices down. What are a few things you can easily do *daily* or weekly as a ritual to set yourself up for success?

For example, setting a timer to remind yourself to drink water, writing your "to-dos" in your calendar the night before, or making a weekly shopping list of your favorite healthy foods.

5. Environment

This is key. Set up your kitchen, workplace, and community to empower the type of goals you want to achieve. How can you stay consistent if you have a lot of junk food around and your gym bag or running shoes are tucked away somewhere?

The better your environment is set up for your health, the greater chance you have of accomplishing short-term and long-term goals. This is sometimes overlooked. Clear out the *roadblocks*. Think ahead!

Does your kitchen, workflow, and community/friends support your goals? Check. You may be surprised. Take a moment and think of potential roadblocks that may get in the way, along with healthy adjustments you could make in your environment to support this.

<u>Here's a bonus:</u>

Once the thoughts above are in place, don't worry about taking anything *out* of your diet, but start by *adding* more fresh, whole, less-processed foods. Think "whole foods" defined as a single ingredient.

This includes all fruits, vegetables, meat, nuts, beans, rice, and the like. By integrating these consistently into your diet over highly processed foods (junk food), you've taken a huge step in prevention from sickness, disease, inflammation, and poor mental health. Make it fun. Mix it up. Explore new foods.

To help start you off, these are five easy ways to apply healthy lifestyle changes to your routine:

1. Plan, prioritize, and prepare

Make it easy on yourself. Try meal prepping in advance for three days at a time (or a certain meal daily like breakfast), picking up premade meals at your local grocery store, or even try a meal delivery system. There are lots of options out there these days!

Choose what works best for you and your budget. Remember, you can't take healthy action if you're not set up to do it. *This is where action begins.*

2. Quality over quantity

The better quality of food you can choose the better. This has been shown to improve digestion, provide more nutrients, and improve satisfaction.

Also, you can usually eat more while taking in less calories if the food is whole and high quality as opposed to refined and processed. Less is more in this situation.

Think, the more the food in its' natural state the better (organic, non-GMO, no food coloring— focusing on whole, or "single-ingredient" foods that aren't processed).

3. Drink water, silly

What can I say, water makes up around 55 to 60 percent of who you are. But did you know that a large percent of the world is chronically dehydrated? I recommend starting with twelve cups a day for men, and ten cups a day for women. See how it works for you (you may need more or less— depending on body type/activity level).

I know there are some people who don't like plain water. That's ok, let's think creatively. Add lemon. Drink low-calorie tea or carbonated water. Just find what works for you! There's a positive impact to your health if you consistently hydrate.

Did you know proper hydration eases strain on the heart, boosts physical and mental performance, cleanses kidneys, and even helps maintain hormone balance?

4. Eat a salad-a-day

I can't emphasize enough how healthy raw vegetables are for you. They supply you with important fiber and prebiotics to support gut health, which are key to overall health and vitality you can't get in other foods or supplements.

That is why I recommend a salad a day (at least). Get creative, find what you like, and plan to apply it this week. I'm personally big on "hearty" salads, incorporating lean protein, such as fish or boiled eggs and healthy carbs, such as quinoa or black beans.

5. Practice mindful eating

Slow down. Honestly, this is my most difficult practice. In the past, I would tend to eat fast (I always blamed it on not wanting my food to get cold).

Research, however, has found multiple benefits in slowing down, enjoying, and being mindful of every bite. These include better digestion, consuming less, and higher satisfaction after eating (fullness). Are you up for trying it during your next meal? You may just be surprised with the results.

In terms of health and nutrition, we all tend to know during this day and age what is healthy or unhealthy. "Eat more vegetables, less cotton candy. Got it."

In life, we usually know *what* to do, we just don't *do* it. The five steps above will help you take intentional action and stay consistent along the way (the key to long-term health, prevention, and vitality).

Lastly, is the idea of *nutrition* and *self-care*. I see nutrition as a reflection of loving and fueling your body, or in other words, tending to your temple (God's temple). Many of us have a poor relationship with food, but maybe we just need to adjust our perspective. Food is life. It nourishes, supplies, and supports our body to live life to the fullest.

So, you have a choice.

You can love your body in a way that lets you find long-term satisfaction in living your best life for God, or you can overindulge and let the blessing of having food on the table hinder your full potential (in body, mind, and spirit).

Many of us are blessed to have more than enough food on the table, yet, around the world people live day-to-day hoping to just get enough (while others overconsume). I believe we are called to withhold from an indulgent way of life.

Imagine if you began to eat just what you needed to nourish your body and gave the rest to those in need. There would be *change*. There would be *impact*.

There was a saying I always noticed in my kitchen growing up as a kid that stuck with me. It goes something like this,

"Live simply, so others can simply live."

This isn't promoting Christian poverty, but whether you have much or little you live simply with the power to give. As I have said before, this way of life will not be easy, and I am working on this area myself.

However, mature growth as Believers is uncomfortable and in opposition to the ways of the world and human nature. It is up to you to make the conscious choice. Not because you have to, there is *grace*, but because this will allow your greatness to begin to unfold for God's glory—so you can maximize your time on earth and love others fully.

After all, you are called to be the light, exposing darkness with your actions and character.

> Ephesians 5:14-18 AMP, *"For this reason He says, 'Awake, sleeper, And arise from the dead, And Christ will shine [as dawn] upon you and give you light.'*
>
> *Therefore see that you walk carefully [living life with honor, purpose, and courage; shunning those who tolerate and enable evil], not as the unwise, but as wise [sensible, intelligent, discerning people], making the very most of your time [on earth, recognizing and taking advantage of each opportunity and using it with wisdom and diligence], because the days are [filled with] evil.*
>
> *Therefore do not be foolish and thoughtless, but understand and firmly grasp what the will of the Lord is. Do not get drunk with wine, for that is wickedness (corruption, stupidity), but be filled with the [Holy] Spirit and constantly guided by Him."*

We must live a life of awareness and diligence, *discerning* the negative influence all around us, and choosing to be proactive before it is too late because the days are evil.

85

God doesn't need you,

but He wants to use you.

Often, we are pushed and pulled through life, "asleep," not even noticing the poor habits we are building or hindering choices that we are making. Therefore, we must take notice. We must be aware.

This calls for *mindfulness*.

Reflect

What does your ideal, healthy lifestyle look like?

What do you want to improve in your life? How will you do it?

What is one small thing you can do daily to succeed?

Chapter V – Mindfulness

"You will keep in perfect and constant peace the one whose mind is steadfast [that is, committed and focused on You—in both inclination and character], because he trusts and takes refuge in You [with hope and confident expectation]."

Isaiah 26: 3 AMP

What do you think of when you hear the word, *"mindfulness?"* Over the years, I have worked to improve my own. I see the importance of it in everything I do, whether I'm hanging out with family, working, or becoming still to pray. It is something I have begun to integrate into every area of my life.

According to Oxford Dictionary, mindfulness is "a mental state achieved by focusing one's awareness on the present moment." This practice can be integrated into everything you do. I love Brené Brown's description of mindfulness in her best-selling book, *Dare to Lead.* She calls it, *"Paying attention."*

It is simple, yet powerful.

When I started working as a personal trainer in 2014, I noticed something my clients had in common. They were not in-tune with or aware of their own body.

This pattern continued to surface as I began working with sports therapy clients who were in pain or had experienced injury, and even continued to show up in my coaching and nutrition clients.

Most of the time, they were unaware of their posture, poor movement, and/or exactly what they were putting into their bodies through diet (and how it was affecting them). I think it's safe to say, as human beings, we tend to struggle with focus. And so, that's what I want to bring to your attention throughout this chapter. Then I will help you renew your mind.

In addition to adding a consistent cultivation of recovery, exercise, and nutrition to your life, mindfulness is vital. Let's be honest, it's challenging to be in the present moment on any given day. Our world makes it easy to stay distracted. We are constantly bombarded with texts, emails, notifications, commercials, ads, and to-dos. Our focus is constantly being challenged, even worn-down.

This needs to change. We must reclaim our daily focus by conserving energy, concentrating our efforts toward growth, and staying in the moment. For example, notice your posture right now! Are you slouching? (I was)

To start, I've provided my top five tips to encourage daily mindfulness and put you back in charge:

1. Set a daily reminder

> Set a time when you know you are busy to stop, breathe, practice gratitude, or whatever works for you to reset and be in the moment.

> The twenty-first century calls for your attention, constantly pulling you away from peace, thankfulness, and contentment. Use this practice to stop and find peace. *HIS peace* (Isaiah 9:6).

2. Focus on one thing at a time

Most of us juggle tasks throughout the day and feel good about it. Yet, concentrating your focus on one thing at a time can help you not only perform the task better but also enjoy the moment (and with less stress). That could be reading this book, playing with your children, working on a school assignment, or exercising at the gym.

Whatever it is, use your precious time, energy, and focus wisely. Our time on earth is short, so let's make the most of it. *Focus.*

3. Perform a mind–body scan

This technique helps you center yourself, to be in the moment, and build awareness. I like to add this in the morning during my prayer time with God.

You can start at the top of your head, working down to your feet, noticing and relaxing each part of your body as you breathe in-and-out. It may feel funny at first, but this truly works and can help you to relax as it releases the tension you're holding in your body.

If you are experiencing a "block" while scanning, ask yourself, "what am I feeling?" What thoughts or emotions are coming to your mind? Sometimes forgiveness, gratitude or prayer and the like may help you move on; even find healing.

4. Practice active listening

This means to engage in your conversations, not thinking about what you are going to say next but practicing truly hearing whoever is speaking.

Notice the little things, staying in the moment, remembering they are children of God. *Lost or found.* I believe this is the beginning of empathy and compassion; what Jesus walked in daily and produced miracles. It sparks the power of God.

Matthew 20:34 AMP, *"Moved with compassion, Jesus touched their eyes; and immediately they regained their sight and followed Him [as His disciples]."*

5. Meditating on the Word

Set a time to read, meditate, and pray in private, just you and God. It could be first thing in the morning, at night before bed, or even during your lunch break in your car.

When you carve out and make the time it becomes special. It shows intention and diligence, while being a form of worship in and of itself. Practice during your quiet time, shutting off all outside distractions (phone, email, and the like).

This is my favorite mindfulness centered passage you can read while in prayer:

Philippians 4:4-9 NIV, *"Rejoice in the Lord always. I will say it again: Rejoice! Let your gentleness be evident to all. The Lord is near. Do not be anxious about anything, but in every situation, by prayer and petition, with thanksgiving, present your requests to God. And the peace of God, which transcends all understanding, will guard your hearts and your minds in Christ Jesus.*

Finally, brothers and sisters, whatever is true, whatever is noble, whatever is right, whatever is pure, whatever is lovely, whatever is admirable—if anything is excellent or praiseworthy—think about such things. Whatever you have learned or received or heard from me, or seen in me—put it into practice. And the God of peace will be with you."

Just five minutes a day goes a long way, and something is always better than nothing. Meditate on His word and you will find life!

Now, to extend my thoughts on mindfulness, scripture tells us you are called to take every thought captive and to set your mind on the things above. Do not forget, your battle is often in the mind, not against each other.

2 Corinthians 10:5a AMP, *"We are destroying sophisticated arguments and every exalted and proud thing that sets itself up against the [true] knowledge of God, and we are taking every thought and purpose captive to the obedience of Christ..."*

Colossians 3:2 AMP, *"Set your mind and keep focused habitually on the things above [the heavenly things], not on things that are on the earth [which have only temporal value]."*

Ephesians 6:12 AMP, *"For our struggle is not against flesh and blood [contending only with physical opponents], but against the rulers, against the powers, against the world forces of this [present] darkness, against the spiritual forces of wickedness in the heavenly (supernatural) places."*

There is power in the mind, and

what you focus on you empower.

Because of this, you must awaken from the "sleep" of unnecessary stress, unproductive habits, and letting a negative environment control you.

2 Timothy 2:4 AMP, *"No soldier in active service gets entangled in the [ordinary business] affairs of civilian life; [he avoids them] so that he may please the one who enlisted him to serve."*

You are you. Perfectly and wonderfully made through Christ to be the "head and not the tail." I know you may not feel like it all the time, but it's not about how you feel.

Feelings fade.

You were created to do great things beyond your imagination for the kingdom of God, not for yourself, but for others. Imagine the freedom and peace in this if you just believed, even for a moment.

Ephesians 3:20a AMP, *"Now to Him who is able to [carry out His purpose and] do superabundantly more than all that we dare ask or think [infinitely beyond our greatest prayers, hopes, or dreams], according to His power that is at work within us…"*

Now, take a step back and remember your identity.

Deuteronomy 28:13 AMP, *"The LORD will make you the head (leader) and not the tail (follower); and you will be above only, and you will not be beneath, if you listen and pay attention to the commandments of the LORD your God, which I am commanding you today, to observe them carefully."*

Galatians 4:31 AMP, *"So then, believers, we [who are born again—reborn from above—spiritually transformed, renewed, and set apart for His purpose] are not children of a slave woman [the natural], but of the free woman [the supernatural]."*

Galatians 5:1 AMP, *"It was for this freedom that Christ set us free [completely liberating us]; therefore keep standing firm and do not be subject again to a yoke of slavery [which you once removed]."*

What if you took the time to be consistently intentional with your thoughts and actions? What would change if you "paid attention" to every area of life, staying in the moment? How would your life shift if you constantly meditated on the Word of God and the truth of your identity in Christ?

I believe your life would change. Take another moment and imagine yourself mentally stronger, more focused, joyful, and driven: living a life for others, with boldness. This is exactly what the world and the enemy doesn't want.

> *They don't want you walking in constant*
>
> *mindfulness of who you are to God, and the power*
>
> *of freedom that Christ has given you.*

Remember your struggle is not against flesh and blood (Ephesians 6:12). There are things, both seen and unseen, pulling you away from the mind of Christ. You must begin to learn how to recognize and identify these areas in your life.

I remember hearing a sermon by Dan Mohler on Adam and Eve regarding *identity*. Whether you believe this to be a parable or a historical event, it holds meaning and truth. Here is the passage from Genesis 3:1-4 AMP,

> *Now the serpent was more crafty (subtle, skilled in deceit) than any living creature of the field which the LORD God had made. And the serpent (Satan) said to the woman, "Can it really be that God has said, 'You shall not eat from any tree of the garden?'"*
>
> *And the woman said to the serpent, "We may eat fruit from the trees of the garden, except the fruit from the tree which is in the middle of the garden. God said, 'You shall not eat from it nor touch it, otherwise you will die.'"*
>
> *But the serpent said to the woman, "You certainly will not die! For God knows that on the day you eat from it your eyes will be opened [that is, you will have greater awareness], and you will be like God, knowing [the difference between] good and evil."*

Mohler interpreted this passage as the snake (devil) tempting Eve, saying she would have great knowledge and awareness if she ate from the forbidden tree: that she would be like God. Adam and Eve, however, we're already made in the image of God, fully whole and alive, having dominion on this earth (Genesis 1:26-28) and deep relationship with God.

He concluded that since the beginning the devil has been trying to shift your mind, causing you to forget who you are (causing your spirit to die in separation from God) and, in turn, forgetting what you're here on this earth to do: *walk in close relationship to God, while living a life of love and impact.*

The world can often have us stressed and focused on the wrong things, but they don't bring life because they are not Truth. They only feed the flesh and are often derived from fear. *Faith has no fear.* We must re-center and refocus our mind to our true identity and the good things of God by being diligent with our thoughts, remembering who we are as followers of Christ.

Daily.

Having said this, I want to introduce a few practical ways you can apply mindfulness to your life, focusing on the five foundational concepts discussed in this book.

These are more than just concepts. They're *values.* You can't have one without the others for complete, holistic health. This is *Wholeness.*

1. Recovery

How are you feeling today? Are you tired? Happy? Dealing with pain? Stressed? Take a moment and process your emotions.

2. Exercise

When walking outdoors, exercising at the gym, or enjoying your favorite active hobby, are you in the moment? Are you aware of your stride, your posture, your energy levels?

Make a note or set a reminder for your next exercise session and practice mindful movement, taking a break from your "to-do list"— even if it's just for a moment.

3. Nutrition

Are you eating slowly? How does your food taste? What is the texture? Are you hungry? Would you feed what you're eating to a child?

These are just some questions you can ask yourself at each meal. Practice taking a minute to reflect. Mindful eating not only provides the health benefits discussed in Chapter 4 but also allows you to be in the moment with friends and family.

4. Mindfulness

It may be ironic to be mindful about mindfulness; but oh, it's a thing. Are you taking the time to write out your thoughts or journal? To stop and take a deep breath? To stay in the moment and not jump ahead in your tasks?

Do you practice taking every thought and action captive? Take a moment and think of one area you can improve this week.

5. Faith

Do you not know who you are?

As a believer in Jesus Christ, you are a child of God. Forgiven. Grafted into the vine. Adopted into the family. No longer are you forgotten or forsaken. No longer are you alone. No longer are you purposeless.

You now have trustworthy hope in the One whom we call Father. No matter your past, present, or future, you have a righteous all-powerful Father who loves you. Stay mindful of this— the faith and the hope we so carry in our spirit.

Proverbs 18:24b AMP, *"But there is a [true, loving] friend who [is reliable and] sticks closer than a brother."*

Jesus.

Next, we will look closer at the potential of your relationship with God and how *faith* integrates into your wellness. This is the missing piece of true healthcare and for those who are seeking *wholeness*.

Reflect

*How might life change if you started being more
intentional with your thoughts or actions?*

*What specifically would change if you "paid attention"
to every area of life, staying in the moment?*

*How would life shift if you constantly meditated on the
Word of God and the truth of your identity in Him?*

Chapter VI – Faith

Faith is untouchable. No one can steal it, and it cannot rust. It is a gift you don't deserve, but a tangible one you carry in your spirit through the Holy Spirit.

How does this apply to wellness? Well, in every way. As an industry, the fitness, health, and wellness fields have evolved from a single focus of the body (physical) to integrating focus of the mind (mental), but rarely have they touched on the spirit (spiritual). Certainly not a spiritual faith centered in Jesus Christ.

I want to assure you that times are changing.

God wants to pour out His Spirit

into every professional field of this

world, including health care.

I believe without a doubt that you can't have complete health, wellness, and wholeness without *God* at the core of your life. He is what holds everything together.

Colossians 1:16-17 AMP, *"For by Him all things were created in heaven and on earth, [things] visible and invisible, whether thrones or dominions or rulers or authorities; all things were created and exist through Him [that is, by His activity] and for Him.*

And He Himself existed and is before all things, and in Him all things hold together. [His is the controlling, cohesive force of the universe.]"

When the situation isn't for you, but you have this feeling to keep trying. To believe in healing over your life although things look dim. To have peace in times of trial, focusing not on what you see but on the Word of God. To believe that if you continue to persist, you can overcome that addiction. To believe that if God sent Christ… He loves you.

This is faith.

Hebrews 11:1-2 AMP, *"Now faith is the assurance of things hoped for, the conviction of things not seen. For by it the men of old gained approval."*

There is power and healing in this unseen mentality. By incorporating the shield of faith into every aspect of your life you can walk boldly as a Believer, being the example that the world needs *in love*.

You can be the head and not the tail

because God wants a generation He can

partner with for His glory.

Life will not always bring what's expected, and things may not always look the way you want them to, but you are called to walk by faith, not by sight (2 Corinthians 5:7). What if you added prayer to your daily situations, your injury or sickness, to those around you in need, or even into your business? Not only when you felt like it, but in faith according to His Word.

> Ephesians 6:18 AMP, *"With all prayer and petition pray [with specific requests] at all times [on every occasion and in every season] in the Spirit, and with this in view, stay alert with all perseverance and petition [interceding in prayer] for all God's people."*

God wants to saturate every area of your life, yet naturally many of us tend to separate our faith from daily life. Our work. Our health. Our family. Yet, since the beginning, we were called to depend on Him daily, in all we do.

> Colossians 3:15-17 AMP, *"Let the peace of Christ [the inner calm of one who walks daily with Him] be the controlling factor in your hearts [deciding and settling questions that arise]. To this peace indeed you were called as members in one body [of believers].*
>
> *And be thankful [to God always]. Let the [spoken] word of Christ have its home within you [dwelling in your heart and mind—permeating every aspect of your being] as you teach [spiritual things] and admonish and train one another with all wisdom, singing psalms and hymns and spiritual songs with thankfulness in your hearts to God.*
>
> *Whatever you do [no matter what it is] in word or deed, do everything in the name of the Lord Jesus [and in dependence on Him], giving thanks to God the Father through Him."*

The Bible is clear that God is and should be part of EVERY aspect of our life, including our daily lifestyle (Lord knows I need it). This is the key to continual wholeness. We must abide in Him. It's what we were first and foremost created for.

Relationship.

> Deuteronomy 6:5 AMP, *"You shall love the Lord your God with all your heart and mind and will all your soul and with all your strength [your entire being]."*

> Psalm 70:4 AMP, *"May all those who seek You [as life's first priority] rejoice and be glad in You; May those who love Your salvation say continually, 'Let God be magnified!'"*

> James 5:13-15 AMP, *"Is anyone among you suffering? He must pray. Is anyone joyful? He is to sing praises [to God]. Is anyone among you sick? He must call for the elders (spiritual leaders) of the church and they are to pray over him, anointing him with oil in the name of the Lord; and the prayer of faith will restore the one who is sick, and the Lord will raise him up; and if he has committed sins, he will be forgiven."*

These actions come through nothing else but faith. Do you have to live this out? Of course not. You have free will.

However, I am here to empower your best self; to help you maximize your God-given potential so you can give your best in all you do. In other words, living a life of power, love, and freedom no matter the circumstances. This is my goal for you, and all God's people.

Paul wrote, while in prison, Philippians 4:10-12 (AMP),

"I rejoiced greatly in the Lord, that now at last you have renewed your concern for me; indeed, you were concerned about me before, but you had no opportunity to show it.

Not that I speak from [any personal] need, for I have learned to be content [and self-sufficient through Christ, satisfied to the point where I am not disturbed or uneasy] regardless of my circumstances.

I know how to get along and live humbly [in difficult times], and I also know how to enjoy abundance and live in prosperity. In any and every circumstance I have learned the secret [of facing life], whether well-fed or going hungry, whether having an abundance or being in need."

God is what satisfies. You can hide from the Truth or give in, pursuing it with faith, love, and passion. I know He has created you for something great. It's just up to you to trust Him; to lean in. After all, I believe in you, and that's why I've written this book. It's time for you to step into your destiny and impact the world, fully empowered by the love of God.

For Jesus says in Matthew 5:14-16 AMP,

"You are the light of [Christ to] the world. A city set on a hill cannot be hidden; nor does anyone light a lamp and put it under a basket, but on a lampstand, and it gives light to all who are in the house.

Let your light shine before men in such a way that they may see your good deeds and moral excellence, and [recognize and honor and] glorify your Father who is in heaven."

I pray that healing, truth, and clarity be given to you right now, in the name of Jesus Christ.

This is a calling, not a statement.

You are created and destined for much and God loves

you, truly sending His one and only Son to

bring you back home to the Father.

So, I call out the greatness inside of you. You must act now, cutting the distractions you can control and stripping off every weight that slows you down (Hebrews 12:1). Pain, sickness, disease, depression, anxiety, obesity, and the like are not your calling and they must go. They are a distraction to your life that the toxic culture and separation from a relationship with God have created.

The following scriptures define what's on my heart:

1 Peter 2:24 AMP, *"He personally carried our sins in His body on the cross [willingly offering Himself on it, as on an altar of sacrifice], so that we might die to sin [becoming immune from the penalty and power of sin] and live for righteousness; for by His wounds you [who believe] have been healed."*

John 3:16-17 NASB, *"For God so loved the world, that He gave His only begotten Son, that whoever believes in Him shall not perish, but have eternal life. For God did not send the Son into the world to judge the world, but that the world might be saved through Him."*

Romans 8:15 NASB, *"For you have not received a spirit of slavery leading to fear again, but you have received a spirit of adoption as sons by which we cry out, 'Abba! Father!'"*

Through faith in Jesus Christ, you know He has taken your sinful place, and God now calls you "child." Adopted into a son or daughter relationship if you believe.

You are home. The passage in Luke of the lost son exemplifies this. You were lost but now you are found.

Luke 15:11-32 NASB, *And He (Jesus) said, "A man had two sons. The younger of them said to his father, 'Father, give me the share of the estate that falls to me.' So he divided his wealth between them. And not many days later, the younger son gathered everything together and went on a journey into a distant country, and there he squandered his estate with loose living. Now when he had spent everything, a severe famine occurred in that country, and he began to be impoverished.*

So he went and hired himself out to one of the citizens of that country, and he sent him into his fields to feed swine. And he would have gladly filled his stomach with the pods that the swine were eating, and no one was giving anything to him. But when he came to his senses, he said, 'How many of my father's hired men have more than enough bread, but I am dying here with hunger!

I will get up and go to my father, and will say to him, "Father, I have sinned against heaven, and in your sight; I am no longer worthy to be called your son; make me as one of your hired men."'

So he got up and came to his father. But while he was still a long way off, his father saw him and felt compassion for him, and ran and embraced him and kissed him. And the son said to him, 'Father, I have sinned against heaven and in your sight; I am no longer worthy to be called your son.'

But the father said to his slaves, 'Quickly bring out the best robe and put it on him, and put a ring on his hand and sandals on his feet; and bring the fattened calf, kill it, and let us eat and celebrate; for this son of mine was dead and has come to life again; he was lost and has been found.' And they began to celebrate. Now his older son was in the field, and when he came and approached the house, he heard music and dancing. And he summoned one of the servants and began inquiring what these things could be.

And he said to him, 'Your brother has come, and your father has killed the fattened calf because he has received him back safe and sound.' But he became angry and was not willing to go in; and his father came out and began pleading with him.

But he answered and said to his father, 'Look! For so many years I have been serving you and I have never neglected a command of yours; and yet you have never given me a young goat, so that I might celebrate with my friends; but when this son of yours came, who has devoured your wealth with prostitutes, you killed the fattened calf for him.'

And he said to him, 'Son, you have always been with me, and all that is mine is yours. But we had to celebrate and rejoice, for this brother of yours was dead and has begun to live, and was lost and has been found.'"

I hear the Father saying, *"You were made for me."*

You. Were. Made. For. Me.

You were made to be a child again, the way it used to be, trusting and abiding in God, able to rest in the truth and the love of the presence the Father brings. You were made to walk in the garden, being guided and taught by Him daily. Everyone can experience the gift of a relationship with God now through Jesus Christ.

Galatians 4:4-5 AMP, *"But when [in God's plan] the proper time had fully come, God sent His Son, born of a woman, born under the [regulations of the] Law, so that He might redeem and liberate those who were under the Law, that we [who believe] might be adopted as sons [as God's children with all rights as fully grown members of a family]."*

If followed and integrated correctly over time, the values of this book will empower you to be your best self. Not in the cliché way people market these days, but fully empowered to fully focus on loving God and others— what we were created for.

I pray that at least one chapter so far has spoken to you and encourages change. Finally, as we put all of this together, I will challenge you to think holistically by integrating the five values (Recovery, Exercise, Nutrition, Mindfulness, and Faith) into your Body, Mind, and Spirit.

Reflect

How might life change if you added prayer

(with faith) to your daily situations?

What if you walked with the mindset that God is good and has

your back in all situations, no matter what happens?

What are you hoping or contending for,

yet haven't asked God?

Chapter VII - Body, Mind, and Spirit

"For those who are living according to the flesh set their minds on the things of the flesh [which gratify the body], but those who are living according to the Spirit, [set their minds on] the things of the Spirit [His will and purpose]."

Romans 8:5 AMP

So, how can you begin to integrate all of this? Let's start with the definitions.

According to the Oxford Dictionary: The Body is *"the physical structure of a person or an animal, including the bones, flesh, and organs."* One could say it's our physical person and what we host on this earth.

The Mind is *"the element of a person that enables them to be aware of the world and their experiences, to think, and to feel; the faculty of consciousness and thought."* One could say it's what we use to act, experience, and view the world as we know it.

The Spirit is *"the nonphysical part of a person which is the seat of emotions and character; the soul."* It's meant to be a reflection of God (we are created in His image to reflect His character, Genesis 1:26) and makes us the unique person we are.

The purpose of this chapter and why I want to bring the Spirit and soul into the mix of wellness is, if we're not careful, we may continue to separate them from our daily life and habits. As you can already begin to see, one part of us does affect the other. Let's continue bringing clarity to the topic.

Here's a visual of how they can relate to one another:

Body, Mind, and Spirit

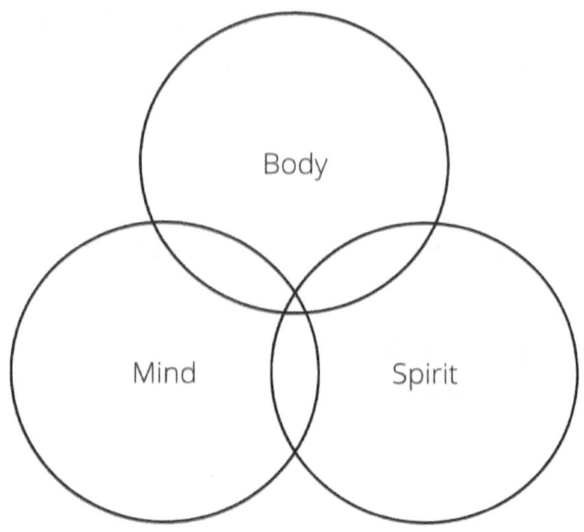

The picture above has been a clear vision of mine for a few years. Now, do you see the very center? I believe when you unite purity in these three areas of your life, "you will see clearly."

In the purity of the body, mind,

and spirit, we see clearest.

In Matthew 5:8 AMP Jesus states,

> *"Blessed [anticipating God's presence, spiritually mature] are the pure in heart [those with integrity, moral courage, and godly character], for they will see God."*

The Greek word *"see"* (horao) used in the Bible expands to the meaning, *"to see with the eyes, to see with the mind, to perceive, to know, and become acquainted with by experience, to experience."* Also, another word for the *"face"* (paniym) of God in Hebrew is *"presence"* or *"wholeness of being."*

And so, it seems that purity goes a long way.

When these dimensions of your self are pure and tended to, I believe (and have experienced myself) hearing, sensing, and loving God is at its easiest. There are no distractions.

There is nothing separating you from

the goodness of, and sensitivity to,

the presence of God.

Even if you aren't "perfect" in doing so (we don't live by works), God knows your heart and sees when you try with honest intention. There is grace.

In addition, there is also an opportunity for you here as an act of worship (Romans 12:1). By intentionally setting the flesh aside, you can begin optimizing areas of your life for Him; to be transformed more and more daily into the image of Christ.

Imagine if you walked with this burning passion? If you walked with this conviction to tend to your body, mind, and spirit in a way that reflects how much He loves you, even cherishes you.

I believe you would operate with power and holiness through the Holy Spirit to a degree you've never experienced. You would see clearly what God has in store for you and walk-in a pure, unadulterated love that does not seek its' own. Daily. We all have a powerful opportunity here. And it's based in self-denial.

Yet, I understand this is naturally what we don't want to hear. Indulgence is natural and a comforter, a form of protection from pain or discomfort (physical, and emotional).

But you have been crafted by God, for God.

Let yourself never forget that.

So, let's get more practical. How can you begin to walk this out? How can you restore what has been lost?

You must remember, you are ever connected as part of humanity, and even more interconnected as an individual person. It's complex and amazing how one part of you affects the other. Your posture can affect your mind and how you feel. Actions affect your thoughts, and your thoughts affect your actions. It's a never-ending cycle.

Because of this, I will touch back on the example of sugar (because it's a good one). If you eat sugar, you now know from Chapter 4 it can affect the chemicals in your brain and influence your mind. If your mind is affected, your body and spirit can be affected. Then as you carry on, your choices, behavior, and even your mood, can be influenced, which you may not even realize in the moment.

It's so subtle. Many of us don't even know

what it's like to feel our best.

Please, don't miss this: there is always a chain reaction. The actions you take hours, days, even weeks before can dictate how you make current, daily choices. For many, over time, even anxiety or depression can begin to sink in when the actions we take aren't rooted with health or Christ in mind.

This all works together, even integrating into your spirit, which I believe can in-turn limit your true potential to love God and impact others wholeheartedly. To make it plain and simple, you can come to a place of not consistently walking in the Spirit as we are called to (Ephesians 4:22-23, Ephesians 6:18, Galatians 5:25)— which unfortunately has become normalized.

Romans 12:10-11 AMP, *"Be devoted to one another with [authentic] brotherly affection [as members of one family], give preference to one another in honor; never lagging behind in diligence; aglow in the Spirit, enthusiastically serving the Lord..."*

At the very least, poor health choices can cause inconsistency, which is the root of unproductivity for the Kingdom and the enemy's main goal (extinguishing the Gospel and the love of God).

As a Believer, you are saved by grace, and the devil knows that. He has lost. All the enemy can do now is slow you down, burn you out, and/or distract you, keeping you focused on yourself. He can get you to a place where it's always about what you're doing, how you're feeling, what you want, and what you need. Yet, Jesus didn't preach this kind of focus on self.

He preached quite the opposite.

> Matthew 16:24 AMP, *"Then Jesus said to His disciples, 'If anyone wishes to follow Me [as My disciple], he must deny himself [set aside selfish interests], and take up his cross [expressing a willingness to endure whatever may come] and follow Me [believing in Me, conforming to My example in living and, if need be, suffering or perhaps dying because of faith in Me].'"*

Remember the revelation I had?

"If everything is a choice, including loving God,

then eating foods that hinder our choices

probably isn't a good idea."

As I talked about in Chapter 4, these choices can include drinking, social media, and other habits that undermine your physical, mental, and spiritual health. We must gain awareness while learning moderation because unnecessary pain, sickness, depression, and the like can throw us off track.

However, when we are stable, consistent, and working toward health in our physical body and mind, we will be better equipped to seek God and relationships with others with clarity, intention, and love. This in turn feeds into the spirit.

Are you starting to see the connection? What if we learned to reset and refocus our lives around this holistic health as a priority?

This may help fuel your spirit

rather than diminish it.

The following concept will help you practically integrate this into your life. In his book, *The Power of Less,* Leo Babauta writes about <u>Most Important Tasks</u> (or MITs). This includes two to four tasks you accomplish first thing in the morning to start your day off right. When you accomplish these, as Babauta says himself, "no matter what, every day is a good day."

I came up with an application you can do daily, working to tend to each area of your body, mind, and spirit. This is meant to be simple, easy, and doable to promote consistency!

Daily MITs

Body:

Exercise with a thirty-minute circuit workout (Say, Corrective Circuit Training from Chapter 3?).

Mind:

Take the time to breathe and practice being still with five-minutes of "box breathing."

Spirit:

Worship or pray and meditate on the Word of God in the *secret place* for ten-minutes.

What's amazing is all of this can be done in one hour or less. What if you consistently started every day like this? How would your life change?

Visualize yourself walking in focus, freedom, health, and intention daily. You have the capability, and I will continue to reiterate, it starts with this foundation of wholeness to be at your best.

"Ok," you may say, "But I'm way off track. How do I even begin to get back?" or, "I'm not where I should be physically, mentally, or spiritually."

Boom. On the next page is a five-step protocol I trust will get you back on the path every time.

1. Pray and repent

Most of us think repenting is to cry out and fall on our knees to God, but actually, the Greek word in the Bible for repent is "metanoia," meaning *"a change of mind"* (thus a change in your direction).

As small as they may be, you must acknowledge your faults and choices that have separated you from God's hopeful lifestyle for you and repent. You can "change your mind" to follow and trust Him, cutting out the distractions, and getting back on the path if you want to. The choice is yours.

Ask for help. He will guide you. He is with you.

2. Practice self-compassion

We are all tempted. We all stumble. Be thankful for your awareness to recognize the roadblocks in your life and receive His sufficient *grace*.

The fact that you care is already a win! Just keep moving forward. Use this time to learn and grow from the experience. Remember the word I had from God, *"You. Were. Made. For. Me."*

"There is no such thing as failure, only feedback."

– John Berardi, Precision Nutrition

3. Take a small action

Easy does it. You don't have to solve the problem in one day. The best way to get back on track is to take a small action toward your goals.

It could be as simple as taking one minute to breathe and reset. *Any small action toward your goals will create momentum and motivation, leading you to change.* You've got this!

4. Set daily reminders

Once you are on a positive path, keep yourself reminded. Set up "triggers," or reminders to keep you on track and stay focused on the goal at hand.

It could be a sticky note on your car dashboard, a daily phone reminder, or even writing your vision on the bathroom mirror. *Whatever will help you remember who and whose you are, where you are going, and to stay focused through the process.*

5. Reach out and find support

Community is essential. *You were built for it.* It's important to let your family, friends, colleagues, pastor, and/or coach know your goals. Ask them to help you and support you along the way.

"Asking for help doesn't mean you are weak,

it's actually been shown to build trust."

– Brené Brown, *Dare to Lead*

If you follow this five-step process, I promise success over time. Don't give up. Failure happens. It's what makes us human. The question is, what will you do from there?

Just keep moving forward. Never forget you are here on Earth to love God and to reflect that love to others. You must engage with your wellness, cutting out distractions to maximize your potential. In times like this, you have a great opportunity to manifest God in all you do, using the gifts you have been given for His glory and helping others. You can be the rock the world so desperately needs through Jesus Christ.

We each have a role to play, but will you commit?

> Ephesians 5:15-16 AMP, *"Therefore see that you walk carefully [living life with honor, purpose, and courage; shunning those who tolerate and enable evil], not as the unwise, but as wise [sensible, intelligent, discerning people], making the very most of your time [on earth, recognizing and taking advantage of each opportunity and using it with wisdom and diligence], because the days are [filled with] evil."*

It all starts with you. Your best. Your selfless best: by walking in the health and the freedom of knowing who you are, and what you are on earth to accomplish. I'm talking about leading your sphere of influence wherever God has planted you and trusting in the process.

You can't always control the pain, sickness, and disease in your life and in the world, but you can do your best to *prevent* them and sow good seed. Beyond that, you must simply trust the will of God through faith, whether for *healing* or for *growth*.

Galatians 6:7-8 AMP, *"Do not be deceived, God is not mocked; for whatever a man sows, this he will also reap. For the one who sows to his own flesh will from the flesh reap corruption, but the one who sows to the Spirit will from the Spirit reap eternal life.*

Let us not lose heart in doing good, for in due time we will reap if we do not grow weary. So then, while we have opportunity, let us do good to all people, and especially to those who are of the household of the faith."

You reap what we sow. I believe in miracles. I believe in grace, healing, and the power of God; but sometimes we must ask ourselves, *"should God perform a miracle when I may just need to take better care of my body, mind, or spirit, and sow good seed?"*

Without correction, we learn nothing.

Hebrews 12:4-10 AMP, *"You have not yet struggled to the point of shedding blood in your striving against sin; and you have forgotten the divine word of encouragement which is addressed to you as sons,*

'MY SON, DO NOT MAKE LIGHT OF THE DISCIPLINE OF THE LORD, And do not lose heart and GIVE UP WHEN YOU ARE CORRECTED BY HIM; For the Lord disciplines and CORRECTS THOSE WHOM HE LOVES, And He punishes every son whom He receives and WELCOMES [TO HIS HEART].'

> *You must submit to [correction for the purpose of] discipline; God is dealing with you as with sons; for what son is there whom his father does not discipline? Now if you are exempt from correction and without discipline, in which all [of God's children] share, then you are illegitimate children and not sons [at all].*
>
> *Moreover, we have had earthly fathers who disciplined us, and we submitted and respected them [for training us]; shall we not much more willingly submit to the Father of spirits, and live [by learning from His discipline]?*
>
> *For our earthly fathers disciplined us for only a short time as seemed best to them; but He disciplines us for our good, so that we may share His holiness."*

God loves you too much to allow you to wander blindly off the path as a son or daughter. We can take it personally and live with spite, or we can choose to live with wisdom and thankfulness. *Diligence* and *stewardship* toward the body as a temple goes a long way. I believe this is where good science meets faith.

Regarding holistic prevention, research has shown an active lifestyle and healthy diet are linked to reducing your chance of cancer and other illnesses such as COVID-19, the flu, and similar viruses by supporting a "robust" (well-rounded) immune system.

Then taking things even a notch further by integrating prayer, I believe you can maximize this prevention and protection with the armor of God. *In other words, being offensive in exercising your faith and walking in the Spirit daily under His wings* (Ephesians 6:10-18, Psalm 91:1).

Below is a visual by Precision Nutrition I use as a tool to help clients gain perspective and work through what they can and can't control. What would *you* write in each sphere?

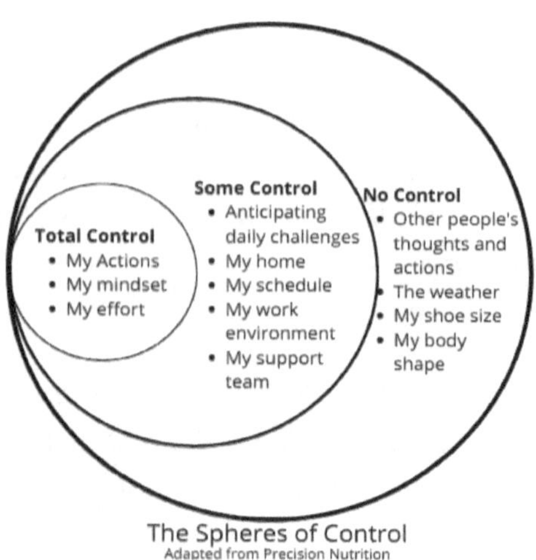

The Spheres of Control
Adapted from Precision Nutrition

I was having a discussion with a friend (shout out to Tyler), and we came up with another *360 Mindset.*

"Control what you can control,

pray for the rest."

All we can control is what we sow. God can be trusted. He is just, good, and a healer, yet there is *correction* and *corruption*. You have free will, and you live in a broken, sinful world. You must not forget there will be many trials, but Christ has overcome them all.

One could say, "we live within the beauty of chaos." And so, I encourage you to take action, trusting and letting God bless the rest in HIS time.

> James 1:2-4 AMP, *"Consider it nothing but joy, my brothers and sisters, whenever you fall into various trials. Be assured that the testing of your faith [through experience] produces endurance [leading to spiritual maturity, and inner peace]. And let endurance have its perfect result and do a thorough work, so that you may be perfect and completely developed [in your faith], lacking in nothing."*

> John 16:33 AMP, *"I have told you these things, so that in Me you may have [perfect] peace. In the world you have tribulation and distress and suffering, but be courageous [be confident, be undaunted, be filled with joy]; I have overcome the world. [My conquest is accomplished, My victory abiding.]"*

You must abide in faith. It is your time to shine in the moments of trial by staying close to God and hearing His word. There's nothing stopping you when you set your needs aside and see trials as an opportunity to exude Jesus.

Let me say, none of us are here by mistake. I wrote the *first edition* of this book during the COVID-19 pandemic and sense that we have a mighty purpose during this time.

You can make the deeper impact this world

needs if you believe in yourself (through Him)

and let your actions reflect that belief.

You can control your choices, your diet, your activity, your recovery, your prayer time, how you respond, how you reach out, and much more.

Now, in order to do this and stay consistent, you must learn rest for your spirit. Which also brings rest to the mind and body. I define this as, "receiving God's love in the secret place, daily."

Rest. This is the foundation of your spirit. Remember "devotional rest" in Chapter 1?

By His grace we can know God's Word (scripture), hear God's word (His voice), and have discernment for what is to come. We are to live by letting His presence dictate our circumstances, giving up our control. Not the other way around, keeping Christ and others from sharing our burdens (Galatians 6:2, Hebrews 4:15).

We must learn to let God be God. The good things come when we let His grace and presence dictate our circumstances, not strive out of our own might. One could even say, strive outside of the Lord's will. I know for myself; I tend to get "ahead" of God.

Here's one of my favorite quotes regarding resting and trusting at the feet of Jesus.

"There is a more excellent way… I'm not going to be *need* conscious, I'm going to be *presence* conscious."

– Damon Thompson, Revivalist

When you seek God's presence and direction over the "solution," things open up for you that may not have otherwise if you had continued to strive and power through a circumstance. Only in *devotional rest* can you accomplish this way of living.

In order to find this kind of rest, and hear His voice clearly, you will need to go into the "secret place." Shut your door. Become privately centered with the Lord and sit down. Listen. Invite His presence.

> Matthew 6:6 AMP, *"But when you pray, go into your most private room, close the door and pray to your Father who is in secret, and your Father who sees [what is done] in secret will reward you."*

Scripture shows us you can walk into the throne room of grace, boldly. He loves you and created you for this very reason: to spend time with you, allowing you to walk in grace and abundance by reflecting His image. Not because you strive but because you are His and rest in that truth daily, no matter what.

> Hebrews 4:15-16 AMP, *"For we do not have a High Priest who is unable to sympathize and understand our weaknesses and temptations, but One who has been tempted [knowing exactly how it feels to be human] in every respect as we are, yet without [committing any] sin.*
>
> *Therefore let us [with privilege] approach the throne of grace [that is, the throne of God's gracious favor] with confidence and without fear, so that we may receive mercy [for our failures] and find [His amazing] grace to help in time of need [an appropriate blessing, coming just at the right moment]."*

2 Corinthians 3:17-18 AMP, *"Now the Lord is the Spirit, and where the Spirit of the Lord is, there is liberty [emancipation from bondage, true freedom]. And we all, with unveiled face, continually seeing as in a mirror the glory of the Lord, are progressively being transformed into His image from [one degree of] glory to [even more] glory, which comes from the Lord, [who is] the Spirit."*

As an illustration of this principle, let's visit a passage in Luke to remind you how God can work in your life, not by you constantly staying busy, but by devotional rest with the One who made you— allowing *grace* to triumph.

Luke 9:12-17 AMP, *"Now the day was ending, and the twelve [disciples] came and said to Him, 'Send the crowd away, so that they may go into the surrounding villages and countryside and find lodging, and get provisions; because here we are in an isolated place.'*

But He said to them, 'You give them something to eat.' They said, 'We have no more than five loaves and two fish—unless perhaps we go and buy food for all these people.' (For there were about 5,000 men.) And He said to His disciples, 'Have them sit down to eat in groups of about fifty each.' They did so, and had them all sit down.

Then He took the five loaves and the two fish, and He looked up to heaven [and gave thanks] and blessed them, and broke them and kept giving them to the disciples to set before the crowd. They all ate and were [completely] satisfied; and the broken pieces which they had left over were [abundant and were] picked up—twelve baskets full."

The miracle in this passage was birthed from the act of devotional rest. Instead of running to the store, Jesus had them sit down. You only find this kind of fulfillment in the secret place, at the feet of Jesus, resting at the feet of the One we call King.

Giving thanks.

This is a kingdom mentality counterintuitive to the way the world thinks and behaves, fully trusting in God who is your good, good Father.

Let God tend to your spirit, growing and learning to love in His presence, reading the Word and being trained for where He wants you in this world— this is "true rest."

There are people in your life who are there for you, but God is there for you even more so, to an infinite degree (Ephesians 3:18). He promises to ultimately take care of you, and all your righteous needs (Matthew 6:25-34, James 4:3). Sometimes all you have to do is sit down and *receive.*

If you would like to dive deeper in your relationship with God, there's a book called *Secrets of the Secret Place* by Bob Sorge that I recommend. I am just touching on the Secret Place and how it is related to your spirit and wellness, but he takes it much further into how you can seek God and ignite your personal relationship with Him.

On the following page are three practical components I believe make up the Secret Place, just to get you started.

1. Prayer

Practicing gratitude, praying for others according to God's will, and casting your cares on the Lord.

> *"The heartfelt and persistent prayer of a righteous man (believer) can accomplish much [when put into action and made effective by God—it is dynamic and can have tremendous power]."*
>
> James 5:16b AMP

2. Reading Scripture

Meditating (or slowing down, mindfully reading and taking every word into consideration) on the Word of God.

> *"This Book of the Law shall not depart from your mouth, but you shall read [and meditate on] it day and night, so that you may be careful to do [everything] in accordance with all that is written in it; for then you will make your way prosperous, and then you will be successful."*
>
> Joshua 1:8 AMP

3. Waiting on the Lord

Resting and listening to what God is saying during your season. Seeking direction, clarity, love, and hope from the Father.

"But those who wait for the Lord [who expect, look for, and hope in Him] Will gain new strength and renew their power; They will lift up their wings [and rise up close to God] like eagles [rising toward the sun]; They will run and not become weary, They will walk and not grow tired."

Isaiah 40:31 AMP

These three actions stoke the flame of the Spirit inside of you, igniting passion for the Lord and serving others while bringing true rest to your weary soul, mind, and body.

So, I challenge you today, review your notes taken throughout this book and meditate on them. Pray, seek, and ask God to reveal your purpose and next steps in all of this to you. Remember to be still. *Listen.* He longs to spend time with you and reveal His wisdom. Without true rest, this cannot happen.

James 1:5 AMP, *"If any of you lacks wisdom [to guide him through a decision or circumstance], he is to ask of [our benevolent] God, who gives to everyone generously and without rebuke or blame, and it will be given to him."*

I know that often it can be scary asking and hearing from the Lord. It may not always be what you want to hear but trust His goodness. Let go of fear. Ask with faith.

I know He will answer!

Reflect

Out of the Body, Mind, and Spirit is there an area of your life you find yourself neglecting more than the others?

What can you do to strengthen it?

How could you implement this in your everyday life?

Conclusion

"Therefore, since Christ suffered in the flesh [and died for us], arm yourselves [like warriors] with the same purpose [being willing to suffer for doing what is right and pleasing God], because whoever has suffered in the flesh [being like-minded with Christ] is done with [intentional] sin [having stopped pleasing the world], so that he can no longer spend the rest of his natural life living for human appetites and desires, but [lives] for the will and purpose of God."

1 Peter 4:1-2 AMP

Your potential in God is endless.

Yet, to fully enable growth you must first find your balance in body, mind, and spirit, building a healthy foundation in yourself that others can trust in and look up to as a leader.

We all must continually work toward this consistent foundation of wellness and wholeness to live life to the fullest. Through this, there's a freedom and opportunity for fulfillment like no other. This won't come from doing what's easy. The days are evil, and the world is in opposition to the mind and path of Christ. Only by living against the grain can you break through.

Will you join me?

At the end of the day, this *transformation* through wholeness is about *identity*; remembering who you are, as a child of God first and foremost. There is everlasting life when you lay down your own, for both the present and the life to come.

Matthew 10:39 AMP, *"Whoever finds his life [in this world] will [eventually] lose it [through death], and whoever loses his life [in this world] for My sake will find it [that is, life with Me for all eternity]."*

If you are going to take away one thing from what I've written, I would want you to know you are created for so much more than you may realize.

However, in order to maximize this truth in your life, you will need to apply consistent action toward true health and wellness: integrating the concepts of these pages with self-discipline, persistence, endurance, and faith.

You were made in His image, and the time is now to let Christ shine in every area of your life. The world is crying out for the sons and daughters of God to step into their identity and walk out the true Gospel with love, grace, and power.

It's a life of selfless giving, yet you will find wholeness through the process. I have a burning passion to see all who believe live up to the potential for which they were created!

My heart is revival.

Ephesians 1:18-21 AMP states,

"And [I pray] that the eyes of your heart [the very center and core of your being] may be enlightened [flooded with light by the Holy Spirit], so that you will know and cherish the hope [the divine guarantee, the confident expectation] to which He has called you, the riches of His glorious inheritance in the saints (God's people), and [so that you will begin to know] what the immeasurable and unlimited and surpassing greatness of His [active, spiritual] power is in us who believe.

These are in accordance with the working of His mighty strength which He produced in Christ when He raised Him from the dead and seated Him at His own right hand in the heavenly places, far above all rule and authority and power and dominion [whether angelic or human], and [far above] every name that is named [above every title that can be conferred], not only in this age and world but also in the one to come."

I feel God's heart break over the potential

not lived in every one of us.

No longer can we as a Church continue to neglect the temple of God within and the power we now possess through Christ. We must nurture and tend to ourselves through intentional recovery, exercise, nutrition, and mindfulness, while cultivating and integrating faith to build a foundation of growth and impact.

Wholeness is about hitting every angle, and in this you can maximize your true, God-given potential. The way of living you're called to may not look like the world, but you're called to be different. You're called to impact the world from a different position, centered in Christ, no matter where God has planted you.

You can be a student and have impact. You can be a stay-at-home mother or father and have impact. You can be a leader and struggling with exhaustion and have impact. It's ok. It doesn't matter what you do, it's how you do it that makes a difference.

God wants *burning ones*.

Let those who have ears, hear.

Mark 4:23-25 NASB, *" 'If anyone has ears to hear, let him hear.' And He was saying to them, 'Take care what you listen to. By your standard of measure it will be measured to you; and more will be given you besides. For whoever has, to him more shall be given; and whoever does not have, even what he has shall be taken away from him.' "*

Matthew 11:12-15 NASB, *"From the days of John the Baptist until now the kingdom of heaven suffers violence, and violent men take it by force. For all the prophets and the Law prophesied until John. And if you are willing to accept it, John himself is Elijah who was to come. He who has ears to hear, let him hear."*

Jesus talks about an opportunity here. Will you violently rise to the occasion of wholeheartedness (zealous passion for God), embracing your greatness? Or will you miss out on the life of impact and adventure God has destined you for?

"You can stumble into the grace of God, but

you can't stumble into wholeheartedness."

- Mike Bickle, Founder of International

House of Prayer (IHOP)

You are called to be a doer of the word, not merely a hearer. You are called to love others, seek the will of God, live out the gospel of Christ, and tend to your body as a temple of God.

I urge you to no longer conform to the world, letting it identify you. Instead, cut the distractions, continue to find your identity in Christ, and be the light of the world; one day at a time.

It needs you, and God wants to use you.

James 1:22-24 AMP, *"But prove yourselves doers of the word, and not merely hearers who delude themselves. For if anyone is a hearer of the word and not a doer, he is like a man who looks at his natural face in a mirror; for once he has looked at himself and gone away, he has immediately forgotten what kind of person he was."*

1 Peter 1:4-8 NASB, *"For by these He has granted to us His precious and magnificent promises, so that by them you may become partakers of the divine nature, having escaped the corruption that is in the world by lust.*

Now for this very reason also, applying all diligence, in your faith supply moral excellence, and in your moral excellence, knowledge, and in your knowledge, self-control, and in your self-control, perseverance, and in your perseverance, godliness, and in your godliness, brotherly kindness, and in your brotherly kindness, love.

For if these qualities are yours and are increasing, they render you neither useless nor unfruitful in the true knowledge of our Lord Jesus Christ."

So, find your team, write down your goals, be easy on yourself, enjoy the process, and never forget who you are. You were created for greatness, and it starts now.

I challenge you to share this book with three people you know could benefit from reading these pages. If you decide to try the **21-Day: Dopamine Reset**, I hope you can use the guidelines and encouragement in this book to stay centered in Christ through the "process."

Trust. Listen. Hear.

God wants to speak to you during this time, and I want to see your greatness begin to shine throughout this next season. Don't forget your "5 Whys" in Chapter I – your true reason for reading this book. I pray that by this time, you're able to clearly see the value of recovery, exercise, nutrition, mindfulness, and faith integrated into your life. Meditate, identify, and apply ways you can add true wellness to your life through these.

There is always more to learn and room for growth for those who want to be *great*. See page 139 to help take your next steps toward holistic action. Find what works for you, trust your passions, and stay true to God's love and path for your life.

As a Christian body, it's our time to unite

and encourage one another to pursue this holistic,

faith-based health I call wholeness.

We cannot have revival without unity. I pray for peace and protection over you and your household. Keep moving forward and keep the faith. I truly care for you and believe God will guide your path as you continue to abide in Him. There is hope, healing, and health in this.

God bless.

John 1:2 AMP, *"Beloved, I pray that in every way you may succeed and prosper and be in good health [physically], just as [I know] your soul prospers [spiritually]."*

Reflect

What's your biggest takeaway after reading this book?

If you'd like, share your answer with Jackson by emailing 360wellnessllc@gmail.com or leave him a review on the Amazon and Barns & Noble website to help impact others!

Visit the next page to get instant feedback and draw awareness to your current holistic health. Introducing, my twenty-question assessment on wholeness…

The Wholeness: 100 ™

Please answer the following on how you would currently rate yourself. 1 being worst-case, 5 being best-case.

1. Recovery

    Currently free from pain or injury

    —

    Typical sleep quality (7-9 hours are ideal)

    —

    Live a low stress lifestyle

    —

    Daily Energy

    —

2. Exercise

    Consistent in daily movement

    —

    Motivated to exercise

    —

    Moving well with quality

    —

    Has an exercise plan or schedule

    —

3. Nutrition

Planned, Prepared, and Prioritized to eat healthy (organized)

—

Eats slowly and with self-control

—

Eats a variety of non-processed "whole foods"
(Organic when possible)

—

Drinks plenty of water (10-12 or more 8oz cups per day)

—

4. Mindfulness

Steady emotional balance (no up and down depression or
anxiety)

—

Stays in the moment (focuses on task at hand)

—

Takes time to rest and be thankful for what you do have

—

Practices mindfulness and taking "every thought captive"
(2 Corinthians 10:5)

—

5. Faith

Spends time with God daily (in the "secret place"— not just praying but *resting* and *receiving* in God's love)

——

Currently trusting in the process and at peace

——

Clear of purpose and destiny in life

——

Actively sowing into others (giving, serving, outreach, and/or evangelism)

——

Please take a moment and tally up your complete score. 100 points is the max. To take action today, you can compare and identify low areas to pour into or optimize the strong ones. Healthy change begins now!

_____ Total Score

360 Coaching Question:

If you were to optimize one area of your health in
this season, what would your next step be?

THANK YOU SO MUCH FOR READING...

YOU WERE CREATED FOR GREATNESS

If this content helped you in any way,

Please leave an online review on Amazon or Barnes & Noble and help more readers discover their greatness.

About The Author

"God has hope, healing, and revival for every one of us. I want to share that through what I do to see others heal and rise from the ashes, shining in this world they were created to impact for His glory."

– Jackson Hale

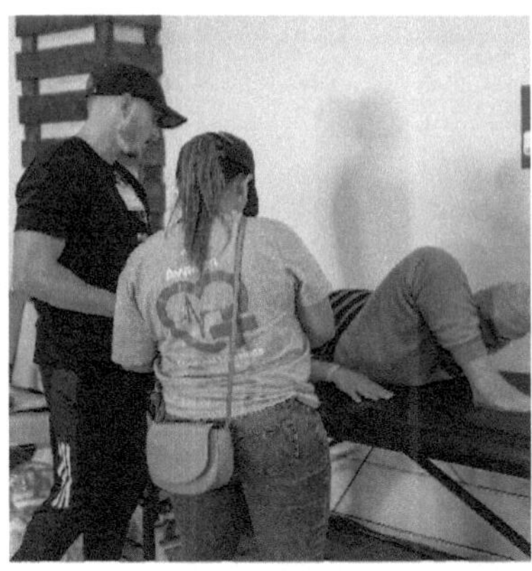

The heart of 360wellness is REVIVAL. The revival of God's people and all who will come to step into all the health, wholeness, and purpose that God has for them. We do this through the avenue of holistic healthcare, integrating practical wellness such as physical therapy or functional nutrition and biblical practices such as prayer or counsel to heal and support not just the body, but even the mind and the spirit of those who need it most. With a background in physical therapy, corrective exercise, holistic nutrition, behavior change psychology, and a passion to change the health care industry our founder Jackson Hale created his own path in 2016. He had the vision to start a new concept of healthcare for "the Body of Christ and all who come."

The core values of this ministry are integrated into everything that he does. These include Recovery, Exercise, Nutrition, Mindfulness, and Faith, making up what Jackson calls "true wellness." With this system, he aims to make a global impact one day by restoring, equipping, and training others to use the greatness they have been given through relationship with God.

www.ingramcontent.com/pod-product-compliance
Lightning Source LLC
Chambersburg PA
CBHW021405150726
47989CB00005B/2408